Practical Medical Ethics

Practical Medical Ethics

Alastair Campbell

Grant Gillett

Gareth Jones

Auckland
OXFORD UNIVERSITY PRESS
Melbourne   Oxford   New York

Oxford University Press

Oxford University Press, Walton Street, Oxford OX2 6DP

OXFORD   NEW YORK   TORONTO
DELHI   BOMBAY   CALCUTTA   MADRAS   KARACHI
PETALING JAYA   SINGAPORE   HONG KONG   TOKYO
NAIROBI   DAR ES SALAAM   CAPE TOWN
MELBOURNE   AUCKLAND
and associated companies in
BERLIN   IBADAN

Oxford is a trade mark of Oxford University Press

First published 1992
© Alastair Campbell, Grant Gillett, Gareth Jones 1992

ISBN 0 19 558234 9

Cover design by Chris O'Brien
Photoset in Bembo by Computype Ltd Auckland
and printed in Hong Kong
Published by Oxford University Press
1A Matai Road, Greenlane, Auckland 5, New Zealand

Contents

Authors

Alastair V. Campbell is Professor of Biomedical Ethics and Director of the Bioethics Research Centre, Medical School, University of Otago in Dunedin. A graduate of Edinburgh University (MA, BD) and of San Francisco Theological Seminary (ThD) he spent 20 years as a teacher of theology in Edinburgh prior to taking up his current post. He was the Founding Editor of the *Journal of Medical Ethics* and is the author of eight books and numerous articles on pastoral care and counselling, and on medical ethics. He is Chairperson of the Otago Area Health Board Ethics Committee and a member of the Health Research Council Ethics Committee. His publications include *Moral Dilemmas in Medicine* (3rd edn 1984), *Rediscovering Pastoral Care* (2nd edn 1986), and (with R. Higgs) *In That Case: Medical Ethics in Everyday Practice* (1985).

Grant Gillett is a consultant neurosurgeon for the Otago Area Health Board and Senior Lecturer in Medical Ethics. He trained in medicine at Auckland University, then did his specialist training there, culminating in a Fellowship of the Royal Australasian College of Surgeons. He did a Doctorate in Philosophy at Oxford University, specializing in medical ethics. He is the first Commonwealth appointee to a Medical School post in medical ethics at the University of Otago. He is the author of *Reasonable Care* (Bristol Press, England) and *Representation, Meaning and Thought* (Oxford University Press, England). He has consulted on ethics to the New Zealand Health Department and was principal author for the B.M.A. report on euthanasia which was released in 1988 in London. He is involved in work with ethics committees and interest groups throughout New Zealand.

D. Gareth Jones has been Professor of Anatomy and Chairman of the Department of Anatomy at the University of Otago since 1983. Prior to this he held positions in the Anatomy Departments at the University of Western Australia and University College, London. He is also Director of the Neurosciences Research Centre at the University of Otago. In addition to his neurobiological research interests in the plasticity of nerve cells and synaptic connections, he has a long-standing interest in ethical issues, particularly in the areas of reproduction, embryology, and neurobiology. He has published extensively in the neurosciences and in bioethics, including *Brave New People: Ethical Issues at the Commencement of Life* (1984), *Manufacturing Humans: The Challenge of the New Reproductive Technologies* (1987), and *Brain Grafts: Parkinson's Disease, Fetuses and Ethics* (1989).

Preface

As its title implies, this is intended to be a practical book, one which will be of immediate relevance to health-care professionals and to the users of health services. We believe that medical ethics arises from the dilemmas of everyday practice and that it must return to specific cases, after a period of critical reflection about one's own views and the views of others.

Thus, although we leave it to people to make up their own minds on the many contentious issues in medical ethics, we do not shrink from offering our own conclusions, backed by what we consider to be the more convincing arguments. This (we hope) will give our readers something to react to, either in agreement or disagreement, and so to decide how to approach the dilemmas they will face. A purely speculative medical ethics is, in our view, a rather pointless exercise.

It will be clear that we have a particular readership primarily in mind in this volume – medical students and medical practitioners at all stages of their careers. We emphatically do *not* believe that 'medical ethics is only for doctors', and we hope to attract a wide readership from outside the medical profession. But — for an entirely practical reason — we have written this book as though we were addressing doctors in the first instance. Our reason is that we believe that each health-care profession has particular challenges to meet *and* particular blind spots to overcome. A book addressed in a vague and general way to 'health-care professionals' will easily skim over some of the harder moral issues which specific professional groups must face. Since all three authors are currently employed as teachers of undergraduate medical students, we have taken this as our primary group and have imagined ourselves speaking to the serried rows of medical classes. We hope that this volume will become a basic textbook in the subject for any medical curriculum which includes ethics as a serious and critical component (rather than as optional icing on the cake or bland reassurance for the initiate).

However, although we start on a medical basis, we have an essentially interprofessional and interdisciplinary aim. We have no intention of confining medical ethics to a 'secret' medical domain. Rather, since as well as being members of Otago Medical School we are also members of Otago University Bioethics Research Centre, our approach is based on discussion with colleagues in philosophy, theology, and law, and has gained many insights from professional approaches to health care outside medicine. The more widely this book is read, the more we will have fulfilled our aims in writing it; and we look forward to the debates it may provoke.

Writing as a team of authors is rarely an easy task. We each come from different theoretical backgrounds and personal perspectives, and each have our own style of expression. We have tried as far as possible to find a common language and (since this is a team effort) we have not ascribed specific chapters to individual authors. We have all had a part in the whole book, by means of critical comment on chapters by our fellow authors. In the event, gaining a common approach proved to be easier than we had expected and we hope that the outcome will read as a unified and coherent work.

We wish to record our thanks to those who have assisted us with the editing and collating of the material and preparing the typescript, in particular Barbara Telfer and Christine Cooper.

Alastair Campbell
Grant Gillett
Gareth Jones

Otago Medical School
Dunedin
October 1991

Chapter 1

The foundations of medical ethics

Introduction

Medical ethics is an applied branch of ethics or moral philosophy. It attempts to unravel the rights and wrongs of different areas of health care practice in the light of philosophical analysis.

> Doctor A has a daring theory about leukemia. If he is right, he will save his patients from a burdensome course of treatment because his theory concerns the use of vitamins and diet rather than standard courses of chemotherapy. If he is wrong, the patient stands to die of a potentially treatable disease. The doctor knows that most patients would be quite alarmed if he told them they have leukemia. He does not want them 'hiving off' to other doctors and/or asking a lot of awkward questions about conventional treatment, so he tells them they have some blood cells which are a little disordered in their growth and need extra vitamins and careful watching. He does not tell them that some people would regard their disease as malignant, nor does he explain the risks to their health which might result from his singular approach to the disease. After a few months it becomes apparent that his approach is not working. He admits that he is wrong and goes back to administering conventional methods.

Many of us realize that this doctor has not acted correctly, but when we come to analyse just what is wrong and how one should act in such situations, that realization alone is not enough. It is here that applied moral philosophy makes its contribution.

Ethics itself has a long history; 'It is not a trivial question, Socrates said: What we are talking about is how one should live.' (Williams, 1985). Socrates asks 'What sort of person ought one to be?' and thus relates ethics to personal morality and character. The subject of ethics is best thought of as the critical scrutiny of moral thought and morality as it affects our ideas of right conduct. For instance, we think it is right not to kill, as a matter of moral law, but an ethicist would ask why we think this and whether our conviction of its wrongness is justified when subject to critical scrutiny.

1

Some historical background

Plato answered the ethical question by stating that a good person was one who, in his mind, attended to and was guided by the 'form' of the good. The form of the good was a divine and eternal reality only imperfectly seen in everyday human existence but supremely disclosed by the calm contemplations of a wise man. Some still think of the good in this way, but most of us would look for something more practical and tied to our normal activity. We recognize that great thoughts do not always mean great deeds, and that morality has something essentially to do with our attitudes, behaviour, and relations one to another. Aristotle offered a more pragmatic analysis according to which forms were 'modes' of being actually found in the creatures around us, and the form of human excellence was that form of life which best suited rational social animals (or mortal beings). We could think of excellence of human form as living so as to properly display those qualities which make us human. For Aristotle, these qualities were shown in our thinking, our associations with each other and our functions as members of the natural order.

If we make the leap from Aristotle to Hume, then the 'form' which constitutes right living is taken to be exemplified by decent, clear-thinking eighteenth century gentlemen. Such persons were required to have 'sound sentiments' and thus they had to have some regard for norms with a broader basis than their own good opinions of themselves. However, it was clear to Hume that morals depended on the *sentiments* of decent persons and were, in essence, a matter of emotion. When we translate this into terms suited to medical ethics, we get the image of a decent, kind medical person, with sound opinions. Such a doctor would do what he felt was best for his patients but might not do what they would prefer to have happen to them because he might not understand or share his patient's point of view on a given situation. The problem is that our assessments of what is for the best can vary from sensitive and informed consideration for another person's feelings to a rather arrogant assumption that one knows best, often referred to as 'paternalism'.

The paternalistic doctor makes decisions for others on the basis of what he thinks best according to his own values (which they may not share). Such a doctor, if misguided, can be positively harmful to his patients. Imagine, for instance, an enthusiastic young cardiologist who believes that everybody with chest pain should have a cardiac catheter investigation. In pursuing this policy, he may have little regard for the patient's wishes regarding intervention for heart disease, or for properly informing the patient about the expected risks and benefits of the test being contemplated (indeed, he may not have thought those out properly for himself). This approach ignores what we might regard as proper ethical constraints on medical practice because it tends to equate the right decision with what the doctor feels to be right for the patient. The difficulty with a focus on the character and soundness of the sentiments of the doctor is that it can divert our attention from the fact that it is the patient's interests that have always (since Hippocrates at least) been paramount in medical ethics.

Codes of conduct

A more contemporary version of the ethical question has shifted from character to conduct and asks: 'What should a person do?' or, for medical ethics, 'What should a doctor do?'.

The most forthright answer is contained in Kantian theories: A person should do his duty. In fact, this is a degenerate version of Kant's answer which was that one should act so that, were one to be a member of a community who all acted that way, one would be satisfied. To be sure, he saw the more general imperative as generating a series of specific duties, and it is these that have been picked up in the post-Kantian strands of medical ethics. Kantian ethics focus on rights and duties, and tend to stress the absolute nature of both. Thus, we are told that patients have a right to life or a right to information. We are also told by some that doctors should always save life or always preserve confidences. Some of these rights and duties emerge when one tries to draw up practical guidelines to regulate the conduct of members of a community of different people. Such a conception of rights can be attacked as a purely social creation but this does not square with the idea that we believe that all human beings ought to be treated in ways which count as decent and that therefore any society has an obligation to respect what we might call human rights. But it remains a mystery just where these rights originate when we try to give them a more fundamental basis than societal arrangements (like statutory law), or when they are discussed in an area like patient care where the law may not comment in any detail.

However, the great weakness of Kantian theories is that one can easily produce situations where duties conflict. For instance, surely a doctor has a duty to save life, but consider the following situation.

Agnes, an elderly lady with severe dementia, in fact almost vegetative, is in a rest home (in the actual case this home was called 'The Greenhouse') and suffers a fractured neck of femur, then a paradoxical stroke and pneumonia. As she is dying, a priest visits her to administer the final absolution. He requests that her nasogastric tube be removed while he gives her the wafer, and this is done. Just as he is finishing, the nurse returns and reinserts the tube because it is time for her afternoon feed and it is their duty not to hasten her death. Ten minutes later she dies.

We all realize that something has gone wrong here, and it can fairly readily be attributed to an adherence to absolute duties. The problem is that it is difficult to see what we should put in the place of duties. We get a clue to the fact that we need more than just a list of duties when we have to resolve a conflict between duties. For instance, one is justified in waiving the absolute duty to confidentiality if one learns that a male patient is systematically abusing his infant children. So, how do we decide what is the right thing to do in these cases? Our conceptions of duty cannot help because they merely prescribe specific types of conduct. They do not tell us of any deeper values which can be used to resolve conflicts between them.

We could regard duties as no more than relatively stable rules devised within a more general moral system which takes account of the *effects* or *consequences* of what we do and does so in a special way for those in medical practice. But where does this system originate from and what is its underlying rationale? Such questions have produced an answer which has formed the basis of the other major strand of thinking in medical ethics.

Utilitarian theories

A utilitarian approach rests on the premise that the right thing to do is to create the greatest good for the greatest number. It therefore focuses not on our actions and their accord with our conceptions of duty but on the consequences of those actions. This system generates an obligation to do our best to increase happiness and diminish suffering. This is a very congenial aim for most health care workers who tend to see their profession as involved in benefitting humankind in ways to do with health. However, things are not quite that simple because utilitarianism has problems of its own.

The first concerns how we *measure* the favoured outcomes. With health care interventions this may seem to be easy. However, people differ greatly in their perceptions of what is of value and thus, even in health care, the relevant sum of benefits might not be ascertainable. Even if there were some agreed conception of what, in general, was a good outcome, it soon becomes apparent that the sums are going to be hideously difficult in all but the most simple cases. The things we must compare include not only quantitative differences in outcome – one-year survival versus three – but also qualitative differences between outcomes. Health care ethics has to consider the value of having an adult education versus having a varicose vein operation, or having a short life with cancer versus a longer life in which one might feel unwell and be disabled in certain ways. When we find that microeconomists are sceptical not only about *inter*-personal comparisons of preference and value but about *intra*-personal preference rankings the idea of a useful arithmetic guide to benefit looks not only bleak but hopeless.

Besides this, we have intuitions about goodness and preference which make pure preference-based utilitarianism very suspect. If I lived in Huxley's Brave New World, then I would prefer a life of convenient and shallow hedonistic pleasures to any struggle with the uncertainties of 'normal', uncontrolled and sometimes unpleasant human existence. But most of us regard the fact that I would have been conditioned to enjoy Brave New World from before my birth as morally odious. If it is morally odious, then that is not because it goes against my preferences. In a similar vein, if I were implanted with electrodes in my hypothalamus so that stimulating them caused me great pleasure (which I preferred to anything else whatsoever), then I might perform a socially useful function for a considerable part of my waking life for the sole reward of getting such stimulation. But we have to ask ourselves whether the balding human organism whose sole enjoyment is being electrically stimulated in his brain is living what anyone ought to call a good life (even though he prefers it).

As if this were not enough, we have the 'Christians and lions' problem. Imagine that we had a small minority of Christians and a large majority of bloodthirsty populace who enjoyed seeing people torn apart by lions. When we do the sums, the happiness of the bloodthirsty majority is much bigger than the misery of the victims. It emerges that, on a utilitarian view, we should just throw the Christians to the lions because morality demands it. And morality demands it because it would increase the net happiness in the situation and therefore, overall, be of benefit to our community. A similar neglect of the claims of individuals because of a wider benefit motivates a utilitarian argument for punishing the innocent. If punishment decreases crime, and we want to achieve that good end, then we should ensure we find a criminal for every serious crime, so that the social mythology becomes 'You always get caught'. If this resulted in killing or punishing a few innocent victims, it could still be morally justified by the net deterrent effect and consequent security and contentment in society. Of course, it would have to be a closely guarded secret that some of the convictions were rigged. But this view just cannot be right. Indeed, Elizabeth Anscombe remarks that anyone who thinks that one can seriously ask whether it might be morally justified to execute the innocent as a matter of social policy, is not worth talking to about ethics because he has a corrupt mind (Anscombe, 1981). This practice seems just as wrong as it is to break a promise to a dying patient, or to allow people to examine a woman under general anaesthetic when she has explicitly requested that it not be done. But why are these things wrong if they don't cause any harm to those who are allegedly wronged? Most would answer that they are wrong because they indicate a lack of moral sensitivity and integrity.

Virtue ethics

The evident problems with codes of conduct, or with a monolithic social value like utilitarian benefit, have forced us to reconsider the qualities of character which are expressed by what an agent does. We have focused on moral sensitivity and integrity, and now must ask what it is to be a person of sensitivity and integrity. We might suggest that it is to be a 'person of sound sentiment'. This claim brings us close to what is called *virtue theory*. According to virtue theory, it is character that is the focus of moral concern, and an agent who shows virtues such as kindness, generosity, respect for others, honesty, compassion, and so forth, will be the model of moral conduct.

This appears to bring us full circle in that it suggests that medical ethics rests on the opinions and judgement of health care workers. Thus, we cannot let things rest here. This is too vague and, in any case, even the most vitriolic critics of doctors would accept that most are decent people acting as best they can according to their own lights. Therefore, we have to spell out how a decent person ought to act in the day by day practice of medicine. We need to devise a conception of virtuous practice that does not suggest that a doctor, for instance, can dictate what ought to happen to other people. An experienced health care worker's opinions are, of course, somewhat special as they are informed by and based on scientific knowledge and long experience of clinical problems. Therefore we are not going to be able to get health-care professionals out of a fairly central part of the picture because their experience will be an invaluable asset in weighing up the pros and cons, and likely outcomes of a given situation. Although there may be considerable weight left on the shoulders of doctors and other health-care professionals, we must seek an independent conception of what it is for professionals to act rightly in their clinical lives.

A professional ethic

We are not totally bereft of a guide in our search for a foundation for medical ethics because the Hippocratic oath, despite its archaic terms of reference, is fairly demanding in its requirements on medical practice. It begins with a rather forceful statement about the duties of belonging to a special group and thereby deferring to one's colleagues in that group. This, although it can lead to gross distortions in medical care, is not so bad as it might seem at first pass. We must remember that the context of the oath was one in which a number of practitioners were going about doing things to people, allegedly for the betterment of their health, but without any training or regulation of their practices. If we accept that health care should benefit the patient, then a fundamental feature of the ethical practice of medicine is that we undertake only that care which is well informed by knowledge of what will protect and enhance the health of the patient. That implies that we ought to require a commitment to an accredited and well trained group of professionals by those who presume to deliver health care. Once we have this commitment in place, we can go on to establish a notion of professional integrity so that certain duties and standards apply to what we do.

The first concern of the Hippocratic oath was, it seems, to set apart those individuals prepared to submit to the discipline and standards of medicine. These have, of course, changed a great deal from the days of Hippocrates (so we no longer swear not to use the knife for a stone, and so forth). But the oath reminds us that the *sine qua non* of the ethical analysis of a problem in medicine must be to ask whether the individuals concerned have acted in accordance with adequate standards of medical care. If they have not done that, then they have failed at the starting gate regardless of what else they did. It is under this head that we place those who do not see their patients when they should, who see and treat patients while in an impaired state, or who neglect to act with due care and attention in their professional conduct. In modern medical practice, the standards are both clinical and scientific.

The second feature of the Hippocratic oath is that one ought to act in the best interests of patients, or for their benefit, or 'to keep them from harm and injustice'. Thus, we have a duty to determine what the welfare of the patient requires us to do, and to do it in such a way as to maximize the chances of the patient getting the best possible outcome in terms of her life and purposes. This introduces something that is implicit in best interests, but never stated explicitly in the oath: one ought to find out what the patient actually wants. It is quite legitimate for a patient to say 'Well, thank you doctor, I realize that I have got a cancer in my liver but rather than having all those tests and operations, I would just as soon go home and end my life in peace.' The final arbiter of what is in the patient's best interests is, almost always, the patient. The doctor must always respect and discuss the patient's perspective on his problem.

Autonomy

This brings us to a third feature of good medical care which is again implicit in a broadly Aristotelian approach to patients and their well-being. Patients are individual persons and, as such, have their own opinions and aims in life which require them to act intelligently in most of the things that they do. But in order to act intelligently, the patient must:

a)   be given information; and
b)   be allowed to make up his own mind.

It is incumbent, therefore, on the doctor both to inform her patient about his disease and its management, and to allow him to make those significant choices required where the disease affects the course of his life and career. There is no adamantine right way to manage a health problem in any but the most simple of conditions. Some people have quite particular problems which require careful and sensitive handling if their disease and its sequelae are to be managed so as to serve their best interests. For this reason doctors, and health care professionals in general, must abandon paternalistic attitudes and include their patients as participants in their health care decisions; that is what respect for persons involves.

We should note that this moral consideration assumes what we would properly call autonomy, and not mere wilfulness. This implies a respectful and broadly rational dialogue between doctor and patient, in order to combine the patient's values and the doctor's expertise to produce benefit. For this to happen, both the patient and the doctor must be prepared to listen to one another, think about what is being said, and be responsible about their respective roles. It is clear that this is facilitated in a climate of openness and trust.

A worthwhile life

Regarding people first and foremost as persons, and not just biological entities, has the added implication that there may be situations in which the patient's autonomy and the doctor's beneficence may point away from preserving life.

Persons have their own identities, experiences of life, and abilities to act on things around them. These are basic to formulating their own values and exercising autonomy, and they imply that we ought to respect the values of, or have a moral concern for, the patient as a person. However, these capacities, even though they are not merely biological, depend on biological integrity for their functioning and can be destroyed by, for instance, injury to the brain. This means that the especial moral concern we normally have for a person may not apply to what is, in other respects, a living human body. The idea that there can be kinds of life that are not worth living to a reasonable human being is often used to drive a wedge between the sanctity of life and the quality of life. We shall discuss some of the specific issues arising from this in later chapters but, for the present, we note that our medical assessments of benefit should take a careful account of what will actually or substantially benefit the patient in terms of a quality of life that a reasonable person would appreciate.

This does not mean that we can decide that certain persons are substandard and ought to be disposed of, nor does it mean that we deny treatment to human beings who are less fit than their fellows, nor that we apportion health care on the basis of merit. All that the recognition of the concept of a life worth living entails is that human beings can quite reasonably and with sound moral judgement decide that certain kinds of life and prolongation of life are of no benefit to themselves or anyone else. The admission that such a judgement is possible does not mean that we must take certain actions, such as mercy killing, in those circumstances. It does mean that sometimes a patient's evaluation of outcomes will lead to a reasonable decision not to undertake certain kinds of treatment even where that might be considered by some doctors to be 'life-saving'.

Some principles

We can now articulate some broad principles allowing us to undertake the ethical analysis of a problem in medicine. This may be approached in terms of basic questions to be asked in situations of uncertainty.

(i) *Non-maleficence/beneficence* Which situations are possibly harmful to patients? For instance, if we find that there is a doctor who regularly turns up to see patients in a semi-inebriated state, it is only going to be a matter of time before an error of judgement leads to a serious outcome for one of the unfortunate patients dependent upon him for care. Steps must be taken to ensure that this does not happen (*primum non nocere*).

The reverse of this coin is a notion of substantial benefit. We could define this as follows:

> *An outcome which now or in the future would be regarded by the patient as worthwhile.*

Note that this is patient-centred, and not doctor-centred, although it may take account of the cumulative and communicated expert knowledge of the doctor. Agnes, in our example, suffered the indignity of a nasogastric tube in the ten minutes before her death. This had no chance of meeting any needs which she then or in the future would be glad had been met, therefore the tube was not ethically justified. We should always temper our medical practice to such a norm. An informed patient is, of course, able to insist upon it, but it should always be the basis on which we judge treatment.

(ii)   *Autonomy* At what point in the situation is the patient's status as a person with the power to decide and act in her own best interests threatened? Here, we can imagine a situation involving a disturbed patient who is incapable of acting rationally or of taking reasonable care of herself. We incur an obligation to attempt to remove this threat to the patient's autonomy as a thinking being and to restore her to normal function. But only *that* is our responsibility; it is not to strip her of her status as a person and force her into a pattern of behaviour which we might more easily be able to cope with. (This is particularly relevant to psychiatric patients.) There should be no mandate in the care of a disturbed patient to permanently downgrade her status. For this reason, a periodic review of our justification for treating her as incompetent is ethically demanded of a doctor who acts to override the autonomy of the patient. This also implies that we cannot undertake any so-called therapeutic measures which will cause a patient to become permanently incapable of functioning as a participant in human society with some degree of control over her own life.

Of course, some patients have permanently lost the capacity for autonomous decision making, and choices must be made for them. The importance of autonomy, however, means that we are bound to act in such a situation as we think the patient would have wanted and justify that in some way. A doctor may justify it by saying 'Well that is what I would want if it were me' or, even better, she may validate her own judgement by getting an independent but concerned perspective from someone else, like a relative or friend of the patient, nurse or social worker.

> Beatrice has a lump in her breast. The surgeon advising her does not tell her that the lump is possibly a cancer and he 'jollies her along' with reassurances that 'everything will be fine'. He mentions, but does not explain, the fact that she will need a breast operation. She, predictably, decides not to have the operation and opts not to attend follow-up because the prospect of it alarms her. At no stage is she clearly told about the risks she is running, and the possible outcome she is facing.

This doctor is ethically at fault because he is not treating Beatrice as a responsible person. He is thereby pre-empting her ability to make significant decisions about her own life. Autonomy, information and respect all go together to form the crux of current ethical views of the doctor-patient relationship.

(iii) *Professional integrity* What is the impact of what is done on the practice and profession of medicine? This ethical question is not just a matter of protectionism for a closed profession but is, in fact, an important concern for any society which wants to have good health care. Health care is not just an instant transaction but a growing body of expertise and shared skills. It depends on respectful and collegial relations between health care workers. These are, in fact, vital to good standards of practice in any unit or institution. For instance, we might find that a certain doctor cannot bear criticism or subject his ideas to analysis in any kind of review. He may, as far as one can tell, be a very good clinician but, nevertheless, there is something wrong with his practice of medicine because an essential element of answerability for what he is doing is not being respected. In the long term, this could lead to a drift so that he was no longer treating his patients according to the best standards of medicine and they might well suffer because of it. To forestall this eventuality, we must detect and remedy the distorted collegial relations that have formed so that his practice is assured of a scrutiny beyond his own impressions of it.

(iv) *Justice* Are we discriminating unfairly in the availability and kind of medical care we offer? This could arise if, for example, two people with equal and telling needs for a certain treatment were treated quite differently based on some bias in favour of wealth or race. It does not mean that we will provide a compulsory and uniform standard of medical care to all persons, but rather that we will accept a certain responsibility as a society to treat people, within certain limits, in a fair way. It seems undeniable that a caring society will aim to make a decent minimum of medical care available to all its members so as not to exhibit callousness to the sufferings of those who live within it.

Above and beyond this distribution of resources that a society sees fit to make available for medical care, there might be forms of treatment which are discretionary and available only to those prepared to sacrifice some other good. For such inequity to be just, we need to explore what we consider to be a justified and equitable level of health care, and remain committed to providing it in some principled way. If we care for people regardless of their worth, this should probably be according to need.

The problem with such principles is exactly the problem that we found with rights and duties: they sometimes conflict. In this case, there needs to be an underlying value or ethos. This 'bedrock' of our moral perception would seem to be the realization that we are all reasoning and social beings who have in common certain biological and psychological needs and vulnerabilities, and that, on the basis of the commitments and relationships that bind us together, we should care for one another.

An illustration

We could illustrate and apply these basic principles by returning to the case of the eccentric oncologist with which we began. The principles, in effect, identify the ethical features of the case and the more general lessons that it has to teach.

First, the doctor submitted his patients to a real risk of harm which contravenes our standards of medical practice.

Second, his actions contravened the *autonomy* of his patients in that he did not explain the situation to them. If he had, he might have been able to claim that he was allowing the patients to define their own *best interests* and been mitigated to some extent if some of them opted for the trial of 'treatment' he offered in preference to the unpleasant chemotherapy which is standard for their problem. He cannot claim this mitigation because he neither told them of the risks they were running, nor gave them any indication that there were alternative ways of dealing with the problem to his own approach. To act in such a way, without telling patients, is indefensible and therefore the profession would be ethically bound to attempt to offset the harm that was being done.

In a case like this, some would argue that professional etiquette, which comprises the rules of thumb that preserve and protect collegial relations within the profession, prevents one from interfering with the practice of a colleague. However, etiquette must give way to ethics when a doctor's conduct poses a serious threat to patient welfare and the practice of good medicine.

This case is hypothetical; one can imagine additional features which would have made the doctor's unethical behaviour even more dangerous. The doctor concerned could have obstructed his patients' access to normal advice and care by colleagues who did not agree with his hypothesis. This would contravene by positive commission, and not just omission, the principle that one should do no harm. He could have proclaimed his theory, unsupported and dubious as it was, to those receiving training under his supervision. This would have prejudiced the future practice of medicine by those whom he influenced. He could have refused to submit to any review of his results so that the harm caused by his views would remain undetected and uncorrected. This, again, would have contravened the idea of a collegial profession. That principle and *primum non nocere* would both be threatened if he systematically distorted his data so that the real preventable harm befalling his patients continued and could not be revealed.

What is more, quite apart from what *he* could have done there are a number of ways in which others might have compounded and worsened his errors. His colleagues could have allowed him to treat their patients without warning those patients or informing them of the truth about their disease and so colluded in his offences against the patients' best interests and autonomy. Similar ethical criticisms would apply if his colleagues let his scientific deceptions go unchallenged so that his trial of treatment was able to continue long after its tragic results had become evident, or if they refused to confront him or discipline him when it did become evident that basic ethical matters touching the medical care of his patients were being neglected under the influence of his prejudices. They could have allowed him to treat only those patients dependent upon the institution for their care to 'experiment' on, so that patients were treated differentially according to factors such as socio-economic status or ability to pay. This would violate the principle of justice in health care. Any of these unethical behaviours would have made the situation, in our hypothetical case, even worse.

Ethics and the law

It is obvious that some of the behaviour described above is on the borderline between the unethical and the illegal. The relationship between medical ethics and medical law is subtle. It mirrors the general relationship between the moral intuitions of a community and the laws which regulate that community.

Our moral intuitions cause us to enact certain laws so as to safeguard what we consider important. For instance, we believe that one should be able to live without fear of violence so we have laws against murder, wilfully causing injury, and assault. We also believe that one should have a certain security of private property, so we have laws against fraud and theft. However, we believe that each citizen should assume some responsibility for the welfare of all, so we have tax laws and social welfare laws. Each of these examples illustrates the fact that our laws are shaped by what we believe to be right conduct. (It must be accepted, however, that much law also depends upon unexamined assumptions or conventions, often inherited from the social arrangements of a previous age. Thus, the law requires continuous revision and reform.)

In medicine we have a set of laws which dictate what a medical practitioner can and cannot do. Thus, we have laws which proscribe a doctor assisting a person to die, we have set constraints on the termination of pregnancy, and we demand of doctors that they show due care and skill. These laws encode the standards we have already discussed. But some health care professionals worry about the letter of the law, and whether they will be held guilty for doing what they believe to be correct according to ethical considerations.

> Doctor D was caring for a forty-six-year-old man, Mr E, who had suffered a devastating brain haemorrhage. She spoke to the relatives and was told that he would never have wanted to live in the mute, dependent, bedridden and paralysed state to which he had been reduced. One night Mr E developed a high temperature, and over the next day or so it was clear that he had a severe pneumonia and would die if it was not treated. She felt inclined not to treat it but to give him morphine for his (physiological/reflexive) respiratory distress. However, a colleague, Dr F, said that she had to treat because the law stated that a doctor could in no way withhold the necessaries of life, which included medical treatment required to save the life of the patient (this refers to the New Zealand Crimes Act, section 151).

We must, therefore, ask where we should turn in such a situation.

Laws always have qualifying phrases which allow one to exercise judgement: terms like 'reasonable', 'lawful excuse', 'sufficient', 'disproportionate', and 'unwarranted'. These phrases are applied by the courts in an effort to give substance to the moral convictions of reasonable or common-sense people. Therefore, there are often mitigating provisions which mean that the 'strict letter of the law' is more of a myth than a reality in dealing with clinical practice.

Dr F declined to mention that the section he has quoted qualifies 'omitting to provide' the 'necessaries of life' with the words 'without lawful excuse'. Thus, one is not bound to give such 'necessaries' to the patient. Judging by commonwealth case law, it is likely that this would be interpreted to include those situations where, in the opinion of the doctor, the family, and the other health care professionals involved and in accordance with any known wishes of the patient, no substantial benefit (as defined above) was to be gained by giving the life-saving treatment in question.

Therefore, we can say that ethics not only influences the formulation of the laws governing medical practice, but also influences their interpretation in a given clinical situation. Most of the time, the courts can be expected to take the view that the ethical standards which govern conduct between doctor and patient will be taken as a guide to what can reasonably be expected of a competent practitioner.

Summary and conclusions

It emerges that there are certain foundations on which we can build an outline of medical ethics.

First, our practice ought to be in accord with a *techne* (skilled form of knowledge) or art whose aim is to confer substantial benefit on suffering human beings. This *techne* is governed by an ethic which is committed to restoring and repairing, as far as possible, the form and function of a human being. Any doctor should be able, with sincerity and integrity, to assure his patients that the care they will receive from him is at least as good as (and perhaps better than) that defined by the accepted standards of contemporary medical practice.

Second, we must always treat our patients as persons, involving them in those significant decisions about their care which will affect their lives and well-being. That is why our conception of substantial benefit is and should remain patient-centred. We must be particularly strict on any violation of this principle.

Third, we must safeguard the continuity and standards of medicine, taking care to ensure that what is done and taught is consistent with an ongoing enterprise in service of the welfare of persons. Only by zealous attention to this aspect of our ethical responsibilities can we be sure that what will be offered to patients by our sucessors will be as good as, if not better than, the treatment we are now empowered to offer them.

Fourth, we must practise medicine in the light of our patients' needs without being influenced or prejudiced by factors which have nothing to do with their diseases. Thus, we must act with justice and impartiality ensuring that our care is given in a spirit of compassion and a desire to benefit, rather than being distorted by any other motive or interest.

With these principles in hand and a real sensitivity to the persons and situations that we encounter we are equipped to address the ethical problems of modern medicine in the spirit of (if not with all of the beliefs and limitations of) Hippocrates. In the chapters which follow, we shall look in detail at the general principles outlined in this chapter, relating them to a series of issues within medical practice.

Chapter 2

The healing ethos

Introduction

What is it that makes a person into a medical practitioner? In one way, the answer may seem obvious: it is the learning process spread over six or more years which inculcates the required basic knowledge and skills to qualify for professional registration. However, this is really too simple a view. Like all professional education, medical education is more than simply the passing on of knowledge and the teaching of skills. It is also the transmission of a whole set of attitudes which the profession has acquired over many years, attitudes which are passed on in many subtle ways by the more experienced practitioner as she instructs the novice doctors under her tutelage.

This set of (largely implicit) attitudes may be described as the *ethos* of medicine. The transmission of this ethos begins as soon as the student of anatomy learns to dissect a human cadaver clinically and to put aside those feelings of revulsion which most people would naturally feel when asked to perform such a task (see Chapter 3 below). A kind of emotional hardening has to take place, an attitude which marks out the medical student as a member of a group which has privileged access to the bodies of others, in life and in death. The student must quickly learn ways of coping not only with cadavers, but with the pain, distress, and mutilation associated with serious disease and injury. Yet, paradoxically, the person who learns to distance herself from her emotions in order to be a clinically competent doctor will not necessarily be a good doctor. The healing ethos is one which combines this necessary detachment with a genuine concern for the individual patient, an attitude which requires a degree of empathy and emotional closeness. Only when the medical ethos includes a profound respect for the individuality of each patient will it serve the true purpose of medicine – the health of the patient. Ethos and ethics are not always the same thing, and what has become accepted practice must be open to continual ethical scrutiny to ensure that the needs of the patient are truly served.

In this chapter, we will survey the ethical features of the professional relationship in medicine by considering firstly the general features of the relationship between doctors and patients, and then focusing more specifically on informed consent, confidentiality, and truth telling. In a final section, we will consider relationships between colleagues both within and outside the medical profession as these affect the welfare of patients.

The doctor-patient relationship

He [the physician] would be like God, saviour equally of slaves, of paupers, of rich men, of princes, and to all a brother . . . for we are all brothers.
(Hymn of Serapion)

This quotation from an ancient hymn to the god of healing, Asclepius, illustrates the powerfully religious origins of medicine. In the ancient world, all healers were seen as sharing in the power of God or the gods to overcome evil. Medicine was an ancient craft, and in the West traced its origins to the school of Hippocrates (fifth century BC), in which brotherly allegiance, respect for the gods and commitment to the welfare of all patients were seen to be wholly interdependent. In this regard a sentence from the *Precepts* of Hippocrates is often quoted: 'Where there is love of man there is also love of the art.'

How relevant are these ancient perceptions of doctoring to the modern practice of medicine? It is obvious that medicine is more commonly seen as associated with science than with religion. For example, Pellegrino and Thomasma in *A Philosophical Basis of Medical Practice* describe medicine as 'the most scientific of the humanities and the most humane of the sciences' (Pellegrino and Thomasma, 1981). In a largely secular society, patients and doctors alike are inclined to see the gods as irrelevant to both the science and the art of medicine. Nevertheless, the doctor is often still invested with a godlike authority, and faith in the doctor's ability to diagnose correctly and to prescribe effective treatment can be seen as an important component in the healing process. There is still a power associated with medicine which seems to derive partly from the highly specialized nature of the knowledge required to practise it, and partly from people's need to find some force which will protect them from disease and death.

An assessment of the ethical implications of this trust in the power of medicine requires a careful look at the character of the relationship which is provided in the modern practice of medicine. The danger still inherent in medicine, despite (or perhaps even because of) the rise of medical science, is that the autonomy of patients is ignored and the paternalistic attitude 'doctor knows best' is used to control the situation. Leo Tolstoy has a vivid description of this attitude in his essay *The Death of Ivan Ilyich*:

> The whole procedure followed the lines he expected it would: everything was as it always is. There was the usual period in the waiting room and the important manner assumed by the doctor . . . and the weighty look which implied, You just leave it to us, and we'll arrange matters – we know all about it and can see to it in exactly the same way as we would for any other man (Tolstoy, 1960).

A different model of the medical relationship is required to ensure that patients are treated in a way which respects their individuality and their capacity to make judgements for themselves. With this aim in view, the term 'client' is sometimes substituted for 'patient', and it is argued that the medical relationship is really a form of 'contract' to be fully negotiated by the practitioner and the client. This approach does have some advantages over the old paternalistic model. It may prevent doctors from acting in what they consider to be the 'best interests' of the patient without establishing whether this is in fact what the patient would choose (Veatch, 1981). It can also help the patient think through the implications of treatment, to take responsibility for the health care decisions which are made, to know what to expect from the doctor, and to take action when the contractual obligations have not been honoured.

However, the contractual model has a number of problems. Firstly, the substitution of 'client' for 'patient' is a semantic change of little significance. The term itself does not necessarily convey an equal relationship. (The Latin root – *cliens* – signifies a person under the protection or patronage of a superior.) The use of 'client' in law and social work is no guarantee that these professions act less paternalistically than do doctors. Moreover, 'patient' is a more accurate description of the recipient of medical treatment and care, since it means simply 'the person who is suffering'. Secondly, an emphasis on contract is in danger of ignoring the vulnerability of the patient in many medical situations. It is relatively rare for a person to be in a position to negotiate appropriate treatment, as one would negotiate a business contract. The technicalities are such that we are dependent on the interpretation of the medical practitioner to understand the options. In addition, illness often has a disabling effect on one's capacity to judge between options, to view the situation objectively and to pay attention to all the detail which is provided. The principle *caveat emptor* (let the buyer beware) is a safeguard which people can observe when, for example, they are considering the purchase of 'bargain price' goods. But such a prudent regard for one's own interests is not possible in many medical encounters. There has to be confidence in the goodwill, competence and commitment of the doctor in light of these uncertainties. We often need to seek help, with only the moral trustworthiness of the provider of care to rely on.

For these reasons it has been suggested that 'covenant' is a more appropriate term than 'contract' for the health care relationship (May 1983; Campbell 1984). The advantage of this change in terminology is that it offers a different approach to the medical relationship. Although covenant is closely related to contract, it contains a greater sense of personal commitment, which transcends a careful calculation of individual advantage. The covenant relationship is open ended, a promise to show active concern for the welfare of the other. Thus it seems to be a more accurate reflection of the sense of professional dedication which most health professionals bring to their work. It implies that respect for the patient as a person is more important to the doctor than a constant striving for status, income, and power. Such a view does justice to the religious or humanistic convictions of those who choose medicine out of a sense of vocation and a desire to help those in need.

There are, of course, dangers in the covenant model and it becomes a question of whether these are better risks to accept than the risks of the contractual emphasis. The obvious difficulty is that it may put the doctor in an elevated moral position which seems to suggest some superiority over other professions and occupations and over patients (who are not expected to have an equal covenantal commitment to their doctors). The result can be an over-idealistic portrayal of medical work which obscures the obvious advantages to the practitioner in both social and economic terms. Conversely, the notion of commitment can result in an exploitation of the practitioner, with nothing expected from the patient or society in terms of an active involvement in the promotion of individual or social health. The doctor becomes a 'lone ranger' battling the forces of disability and disease singlehanded. The result can be an over-involved style of practice which fails to encourage the patient to be an active participant in his or her own recovery, and which can lead to a sacrifice of the practitioner's own personal and family life. Moreover, a stress on the moral trustworthiness of the practitioner can be used to justify the kind of paternalistic attitude which sees no need to enlist the patient fully as a partner in the medical relationship. 'You can trust us' can be used as an evasion of proper scrutiny of what actually takes place in medical encounters.

A solution to these difficulties, however, can be found by insisting that one of the professional obligations of the doctor is commitment to an open, truthful and fully co-operative relationship with patients.

Information and consent

Consider the following case:

> A general practitioner is aware that some of the symptoms being presented to him are suggestive of carcinoma of the urinary tract, but obviously this cannot be confirmed or disconfirmed without further tests. What should he say to the patient, in referring him for investigation? Should he mention cancer as a possibility at this stage, or is this creating unnecessary alarm?

In the past, it would have been argued that the best interests of the patient would not be served by sharing with him, at this stage, the medical possibilities. The traditional beneficent approach was to reassure the patient that there was probably nothing to worry about – 'just a few tests to check things out'. The problem with this approach is that it creates a particular relationship between practitioner and patient that is hard to change at a later stage, if things turn out as the practitioner fears. Moreover, it denies a fundamental value within the professional relationship as we have been describing it – the value of honesty or truthfulness.

An open and straightforward sharing of the available information and the steps that are necessary to proceed with the investigation creates instead a co-operative relationship in which the patient is prepared for a later discussion of treatment options, if this is required. If the doctor 'babies' the patient at the outset, it is difficult to change the encounter to a more adult footing later in the process. The doctor in this case could first say something like this: 'I'd like to arrange for you to have some tests to find out what's causing the pain and bleeding. It could be something quite simple and easily remedied, or it could be a more serious problem, in which case we shall want to do something about it as soon as we can.' This statement leaves the patient free to ask further and more detailed questions if he wishes. The doctor has not specifically mentioned cancer as a possibility, but he has left it open for this to be explained if the patient follows through with further questions. When the full information is available from the test results, this opening discussion has prepared the way for a full sharing of the information which is now available. Then, at this stage, the treatment options are discussed with the patient as a partner in the decision-making process and fully informed of the options which are now open to him.

How much information is required in order to ensure that a patient is genuinely consenting to treatment after a careful consideration of the options? A recent report by the New Zealand Medical Council has suggested the following:

> Information must be conveyed to the patient in such detail and in such a manner, using appropriate language, as to ensure that an informed decision can be made by that particular patient. (Medical Council of New Zealand, 1990)

This is really a double criterion: firstly, the nature of the individual patient is a relevant factor; secondly, in order for an 'informed decision' to be made there must be an assessment of what *any* person would wish to know in the circumstances. If we begin with the second criterion, we cannot expect anyone to make a reasoned decision if they are not in full possession of the relevant facts. They need to know what the benefits are from the various treatments which could be offered, and what the corresponding risks (including side-effects) are. They must be told who will be carrying out the treatment, how soon it will be available, and they need to be informed of the likely consequences of not having any treatment. These are the minimum requirements for any discussion of treatment options. Knowledge of the particular patient is used to guide the doctor about how best to convey what can be quite technical and, at times, alarming information. The aim must be to enable the patient to participate in a choice which reflects his or her own values, aims and aspirations, rather than those of the doctor. A patient who then says: 'What do you recommend, doctor?' is expressing her wish to rely on expert advice. This is a perfectly reasonable request, but in this situation the practitioner must be doubly sure that the patient understands what the nature of that advice is. Relying on expert advice does not relieve the patient of responsibility for the decision. For this reason, it is now being suggested that the phrase 'informed consent' should be replaced by some alternative phrase like 'informed choice' or 'informed request', emphasizing the patient's primary role in the process.

In practice, many difficulties will be encountered in trying to achieve informed consent – or 'informed choice'. Because the partnership between patient and doctor will always be an unequal one, it is rarely a totally independent choice by the patient. Only a medically trained person can appreciate the uncertainties and complexities of many treatment options, however much of an effort is made to convey some of these to the patient; and inevitably a doctor will have preferences, which may well differ in emphasis from those of some of her colleagues. Thus, however much we struggle to exclude bias, it has to be said honestly that the choice which the patient makes will often be dependent upon the particular practitioner who describes the options. A doctor who puts faith in one particular form of chemotherapy for cancer, for example, is likely to present it in such a way that his patients see it as the best option. (This is a variation of the well-known phenomenon that patients of Freudian or of Jungian analysts always seem to dream the 'right' kind of dreams for their respective analysts' theories!) A practical solution to undue influence in the obtaining of consent can be found only by encouraging patients to make themselves better informed, by the production of written information sheets on treatment options and by the use of standard treatment protocols to control the aberrant behaviour of the more idiosyncratic practitioners.

In the last analysis, however, there will always remain an element in the doctor-patient relationship which depends upon the trustworthiness and integrity of the doctor. No ethical or legal requirements for informed consent will be effective without the willingness of those who have the knowledge and power to be constantly critical of their own practice and always open to a perception of the needs of individual patients. The covenantal relationship cannot be replaced by some cast-iron contract which will infallibly protect the rights of patients. Moreover, there are many situations in which the capacity of the patient to decide is either impaired or totally absent, and in these circumstances the doctor (in conference with the family) must be trusted to make appropriate decisions on behalf of the patient. Thus, although the old paternalistic attitude in which patients were kept in virtual ignorance must be rejected, there will be many situations in medicine in which the capacity of the *doctor* to make the right treatment choices is still the most important factor. An emphasis on consent, where appropriate and possible, does not remove the need for a profession which will act 'for the patient's good' (Pellegrino and Thomasma, 1988).

Confidentiality

A doctor has two homosexual men as patients, each of whom consults him regularly with symptoms possibly suggestive of the onset of AIDS. One patient agrees to have a blood test and proves to be HIV antibody positive.

He begs the doctor not to inform his partner, fearing that this will mean the end of their relationship. The partner adamantly refuses to have a test, saying that he doesn't want to know if he ever does get AIDS, and that in any case he 'knows how to be careful'. The doctor is also aware that this patient has a number of casual sexual relationships, of both a homosexual and heterosexual nature. Should he inform him that his partner is HIV positive to warn him of the dangers to himself and his other contacts, or must he respect the confidentiality of the information, and hope that 'careful' means no possibility of transmission of the virus?

This case illustrates the complexity of the notion of confidentiality in the medical relationship. There are circumstances in which a doctor's obligation to respect the confidentiality of the information gained about a patient seems to be in direct conflict with his duties to other patients or to the wider society. How is the dilemma to be resolved?

It is important to consider first why confidentiality is regarded as so important in health care relationships. The provision of medical care always involves an invasion of privacy. Without access to the patient's body and to a wide range of personal information about the patient, it is not possible either to achieve an adequate diagnosis or to provide appropriate treatment. This privileged access, however, is justified only because it is to the patient's benefit, and it is only obtained (except in an emergency) if the patient consents to it. Thus the information gained in the medical consultation, although contained in records which are the property of either an individual practitioner or a health board, should normally be used only for purposes which the patient authorizes. Any other use of the information represents an invasion of the privacy of the patient and a breach of the trust which made the patient willing to consult the practitioner in the first place. In other words, confidentiality constitutes an essential element in the therapeutic relationship, and must be regarded as integral to the 'sacred trust' described in the Oath of Hippocrates.

Does this mean that confidentiality is an absolute which can never be outweighed by other moral considerations? Until recently it was viewed in this light, rather on a par with the secrets of the confessional. To do this commits us to a totally individualistic view of medical care. Doctors clearly have some obligations to those around the individual patient, even though the patient is usually given the prime consideration. In circumstances where active harm to others will be caused, the obligation to confidentiality cannot be an absolute. The problem is defining what constitutes 'active harm'. It is already well established that when a patient's medical condition renders him unfit to drive, this information must be passed on to the appropriate authorities if the patient refuses to do it himself (Cole, 1987, p. 23). Sometimes, however, the risk to others is less clearly predictable. The Tarasoff case in the USA (California Supreme Court, 1976) found a psychologist and his employers negligent in their failure to inform the girlfriend of a pyschiatric patient that he was threatening to kill her – a threat he did in fact carry out. This seems to extend the duty to breach confidentiality in an effort to protect others far beyond immediately predictable danger. What of the homosexual man, in the case above, who was in danger of unknowingly passing the AIDS virus widely among his sexual partners? This example is complicated by his explicit statement that he did not wish to know if he was HIV positive. But the requirement to protect others does still apply, and would have to influence the doctor's decision in this case. In simpler cases, where a bisexual infected man is concealing his condition from his female partner, the guideline has now been established that confidentiality can be breached to warn the partner unaware of the risk she is exposed to, if the infected person refuses to pass on the information (see Chapter 9 below). This guideline might be extended to cover the doctor's obligation to attempt some added protection of the unknown partners of his promiscuous patient. The decision is a very hard one since, in order to achieve this somewhat uncertain objective, the doctor would be obliged to override the expressed wishes of *both* of the patients for whom he has direct responsibility.

In most everyday clinical situations, however, the requirement for confidentiality is much more straightforward. It can be understood as an explicit recognition of the respect which a doctor shows for each of her patients as individuals. To respect the privacy of the information is to respect the patient himself and thus to justify the trust which is placed in the doctor, as a person of discretion and sensitivity. Unfortunately both the content of some medical records and the manner in which they are handled often represents a betrayal of that basic trust. (Access to records for research purposes raises different issues, which are discussed in Chapter 6 below.) In a hospital setting especially, notes on patients can be much too readily accessed by individuals who have no direct clinical involvement with the patient, and therefore no right to acquire the personal details contained in the record. Moreover, notes can contain highly subjective and prejudicial comments on patients. If such comments are discovered by the patient, the whole basis of the relationship is undermined.

A young woman patient had presented herself frequently at the surgery of a general practitioner complaining of tiredness and persistent headaches. She had been referred for several specialist consultations, but no reason for her symptoms had been established. On one occasion she had turned up at a casualty department in a severe panic and with hyperventilation tetany, and was discharged with an appointment for a psychiatric consultation at the outpatient clinic. She did not keep this appointment, but returned to her general practitioner for further advice. During that consultation an interruption gave her an opportunity to look at her case file on the doctor's desk. Written in large letters in the front of the file was the following comment: 'Beware, hysterical and manipulative, determined to be unwell.' The patient lodged a complaint against the doctor, and was left with a sense of being humiliated and degraded by the medical profession as a whole.

Whatever the correct assessment of this patient's condition, the doctor showed a total lack of understanding about the nature of confidential medical notes, using them as a cloak for interprofessional communication or as an aide memoir for himself. Notes should always be written in the form of a record of objectively established findings which have been – or will be – shared with the patient, with an appropriate interpretation of the technical details. Rights of access to one's own medical record have now been established. Some institutions may attempt to block access on the doctor's opinion that no point will be served and the patient could be harmed by such access. This kind of barrier is probably not sustainable in the face of legal action by the patient. The shared status of clinical notes reinforces the basic ethical insight that confidentiality has as its prime aim the enabling of an open and safe relationship between doctor and patient.

Truthfulness

Throughout this chapter we have been stressing the special character of the relationship between patient and doctor, a relationship which seeks to make the patient into a partner in the healing endeavour, but which recognizes the inequality created by the sick person's vulnerability and sense of dependence. In order to avoid the paternalism of the past, the interaction between patient and doctor must be characterized by truthfulness on the part of the doctor (but equally by the patient, who cannot be helped if she acts in a deceptive or manipulative way). Truthfulness describes much more than simply the passing on of accurate information. It is expressed in an attitude toward the other person which seeks to create open and mutually respectful communication (Bok, 1980; Higgs, 1985). It is possible to avoid lying to a person and yet disregard truthfulness by concealing facts or creating false impressions. For example, it was common in the recent past to avoid whenever possible the use of the word 'cancer'. Instead, 'wart' or 'growth' might be used, and any diagnosed malignancy would simply not be mentioned, unless the patient asked directly about it. Such subterfuges are now uncommon, largely because the more open attitudes toward cancer have made them ineffective. However, there still remains a considerable hesitation to communicate a bad prognosis to a patient, while at the same time the family may be 'let into the secret'. It is obvious that such devices create a relationship with patients which is deficient in truthfulness, even if no direct lies are told. The argument that this is 'kinder' to patients does not appear to be supported by the facts, since surveys have shown that the vast majority of people would prefer to be told directly what their chances of survival are, rather than being left worrying about the true nature of their condition, and unable to trust those around them to be honest with them.

Are there no situations in which concealment is the preferable moral choice? The so-called 'therapeutic privilege' has been found in at least one legal case to exempt doctors from passing on information when in their judgement it would be therapeutically counter-indicated. There are some clinical situations in which the condition of the patient is so fragile that a full disclosure of all known facts would be overwhelming for them *at that time*. For example, a person in a critical condition after a road accident might ask about the survival of other family members. A temporary concealment of the full facts might be indicated to save the psychological trauma of hearing that someone had died or was also critically ill. The same argument is often used to justify a certain vagueness about the extent of a person's own burns or internal injuries during the critical phase. It should be noted, however, that these are exceptional circumstances which cannot justify a *policy* of concealment of bad prognoses from patients, on the false assumption that it will always jeopardize their chances of recovery. Truthfulness is not the bald communication of facts: it is the kind of sensitivity to individual need which knows that there is a time to speak and a time to remain silent.

Collegial relationships

We must consider finally how relationships between colleagues should be managed in order to serve the primary end of medicine – the health of the patient. 'My colleagues will be my brothers', declares the Hippocratic Oath. This ancient atmosphere of brotherly loyalty lingers on in medicine despite the total change in social circumstances since the Oath was formulated two and a half millennia ago. The 'band of brothers' who followed the Oath of Hippocrates constituted virtually a priestly group within ancient society, and they were bound together by a semi-mystical religious allegiance to Asclepius, the god of healing. Today, the medical profession consists of men and women of widely differing religious beliefs, whose common allegiance is to a Code of Ethics which transcends national boundaries and specific religious affiliations (The Geneva Convention Code of Medical Ethics, see Appendix). The first principle of the Code is: 'The health of my patient will be my first consideration'.

Thus, the doctor owes a first loyalty not to colleagues, but to patients. However, this does not mean that loyalty to colleagues is of no importance. Members of the public often suspect that professions look after their own members to the detriment of patients or clients, or, in the famous phrase of George Bernard Shaw (borrowed by him from Adam Smith), that 'all professions are conspiracies against the laity'. This suspicion is sometimes well founded. Disciplinary and complaints procedures are often painfully slow and not easy for the ordinary member of the public to understand. (See Chapter 11 below for a fuller discussion of this problem.)

Although loyalty within a profession can sometimes work to the disadvantage of patients, especially when it leads to the covering up of the incompetency or impairment of colleagues, it is certainly more than merely a self-serving and protectionist device. Critics of loyalty to colleagues overlook the fact that the most dangerous practitioner is the 'loner' who attempts to work in isolation from colleagues in the field, and without reference to those who hold a different expertise either within the medical disciplines or in other professional disciplines. The provision of health care is demanding, both emotionally and intellectually. In order to work in the best interests of patients every practitioner must learn to share the decision-making process with others, to consider alternative diagnoses and treatment, and to find correction or support when the decisions are especially difficult and uncertain.

To clarify the point further, we must distinguish between etiquette and ethics in collegial relationships. The rules of medical etiquette have tended to create a medical hierarchy in which each consultant is king in his own kingdom and therefore not subject to 'interference' by colleagues, even those of equal rank. In addition, this approach has tended to guard medical territory very carefully, and has resisted encroachment by other disciplines. Great emphasis has been placed on the clinical autonomy of the individual practitioner, and to challenge this autonomy has been seen as, at best, discourteous and, at worst, positively dangerous to the patients for which the practitioner holds ultimate responsibility.

Although it is important that the judgement and experience of a skilled professional be respected and not be subject to ill-informed outside interference, it does not follow that the totally independent professional is the best safeguard of the patient's interests. On the contrary, the complexity of health care interventions demands that the needs of the patient be viewed from a whole range of different perspectives, and in many instances the viewpoint of the nurse or the social worker can provide a much needed corrective to an overly narrow medical view. We, therefore, agree with Hampton that 'clinical freedom is dead'.

Clinical freedom is dead, and no-one need regret its passing. Clinical freedom was the right – some seemed to believe the divine right – of doctors to do whatever in their opinion was best for patients. In the days when investigation was non-existent and treatment as harmless as it was ineffective, the doctor's opinion was all that there was, but now opinion is not good enough. (Hampton, 1983)

The ideal relationships between colleagues, within the medical profession and between health care professionals generally, is one of both mutual support and mutual and honest criticism. The modern professional expects to be accountable, both to colleagues and to the public which grants the profession the privilege of self-regulation. This entails both regular peer review of one's practice and the willingness to review decisions in an interdisciplinary context. The health of patients is often jeopardized by professional imperialism or by interprofessional rivalry. Conversely, when a case conference approach is adopted, with free communication between staff of different grades and varying professions, the patient's needs are much more likely to be perceived and appropriately met.

Conclusion

In this chapter we have sought to describe a 'healing ethos' which will do justice to the range and complexity of modern health care interventions. We have stressed the need for a relationship between patients and doctors which respects the personal nature of the relationship as well as its grounding in the knowledge and skill of the trained professional. We do not believe that patients will be appropriately helped unless their autonomy is fully respected, and this entails improving their capacity for making choices by the provision of full information, and honouring their trust in the profession by maintaining high standards of confidentiality and truthfulness.

The healing ethos is one which must also recognize the vulnerability and inevitable dependency of those who are critically ill and for whom recovery may not be an option. There is an ethics of care which is as important as the ethics of cure, and death need not always be viewed as a medical failure. It is an impoverished medical relationship which can operate only within a scenario of successful cure. The professional relationship described in this chapter is designed to assist both patient and doctor through all the vicissitudes of illness, or in the words of a traditional medical saying: 'To cure sometimes, to relieve often, to comfort always.'

Chapter 3

The human body

Introduction

Although health professionals deal daily with human beings, and therefore with their bodies, the significance of the human body itself can readily be overlooked. This is because we emphasize patients rather than their bodies. Yet there are circumstances under which we need to consider the human body in its own right. This is particularly evident when dealing with a dead body, and when confronted by decisions regarding what should or should not be done to a dead body. Similar considerations also arise when dealing with living people who wish to donate organs (such as a kidney), since this is an act that may have repercussions for the future functioning of their bodies. We need to consider, therefore, what we think of the human body, what value we place upon it, and in what ways we should respect it.

In this chapter, emphasis will be placed on the dead body (cadaver), since a large number of ethical issues centre on society's view of the dead body. However, we shall not confine our attention to the dead body, since any conclusions arrived at regarding our treatment of the dead body may well help us with decisions regarding the way in which the living body should be treated under some circumstances.

An instructive place to start considering our reactions to the dead body is with our reactions as medical students to dissection. How did we respond on first seeing a dead body (even if that was a 'fixed' and preserved body in a dissecting room)? How do we respond now? Perhaps we find that some features of dead bodies are more significant for our response than others; features such as the face, the hands, or the genitals. Is this because these are the features of bodies that remind us that they really are (or really were) people, and that these bodies were once just like us — living people who did things, had goals and purposes in life, related to other people, and meant something to other people.

The notion from which we cannot escape is that dead bodies are both very much like us, and are also very different from us. They are

31

sufficiently like us to be recognizable, both as human beings and as individuals. Yet they are sufficiently unlike us to leave us with the distinct impression that they now belong to a different category of being from the one we belong to. After all, they cannot respond to us, neither can they speak or move or communicate. We expect them to be the sort of beings we are, but they fail, and in a sense let us down. What, then, is the relationship between the dead body and the person who was once associated with that body? The query behind this is very eloquently brought out in this extract from Nicholas Wolsterstorff's book *Lament for a Son*.

> Born on a snowy night in New Haven, he died twenty-five years later on a snowy slope in Kaisergebirger. Tenderly we laid him in warm June earth. Willows were releasing their seeds of puffy white, blanketing the ground. I catch myself: Was it *him* we laid in the earth? I had touched his cheek. Its cold still hardness pushed me back. Death, I knew was cold. And death was still. But nobody had mentioned that all the softness went out. His spirit had departed and taken along the warmth and activity and, yes, the softness. He was gone. 'Eric, where are you?' But I am not very good at separating a person from body. Maybe that comes with practice. The red hair, the dimples, the chipmunky look — that *was* Eric. (Wolsterstorff, 1978)

The relationship between a person and that person's body is one of the questions philosophers frequently deal with. It is an issue that permeates all thinking about the significance of the human body, and the way in which the question is answered has important repercussions for the way in which we actually respond to dead bodies, both of someone we have known, and of others. As such, it is relevant for medical ethics when decisions have to be made, for example, about using organs from those killed in road accidents.

Before we turn to such general ethical issues, we should consider further the cadavers medical students study and dissect in the dissecting room. This is an activity that, itself, raises a number of issues concerning whether bodies should be dissected and whether prosections (dissections of specific regions of cadavers) should be prepared for display in museums. These are important ethical issues, since the process of dissection involves the dismemberment of a corpse, and this is something society does not allow people in general to do.

Dissection depersonalizes the body. After all, we don't respond to a dissected arm, or even a dissected head, in the same way as we respond to the whole body. What this is telling us is that we associate a person with their body — more or less as a whole — but not with their dismembered arms or legs or liver. Even when we look at a horrific scene (as in pictures of road accidents), part of the horror probably stems from our knowing that a dismembered arm once belonged to a particular body; in a way, we still associate it with a person and that person's body. As dissection proceeds, it becomes increasingly difficult to think any longer of the cadaver as a whole, until it becomes virtually impossible to think of the fragmented remains of the cadaver as a person. In other words, our analysis and dissection have robbed the cadaver of its personal associations.

Herein lies a danger. From this, it is easy to conclude that the reductionism of dissection gives us a warrant to do what we like with dismembered hands, kidneys or brains, even if we wouldn't contemplate acting in this manner towards intact cadavers. Such a *laissez-faire* attitude towards the dismembered remains of cadavers only becomes possible when we deny the relationship they once had with the bodies of living people. As long as there is awareness of this relationship, limits will be placed on how the remains of people are to be treated, and this means the introduction of ethical constraints (including the necessity of obtaining informed consent for the use of body parts).

This is not all. Even the way in which bodies are obtained for dissection is accompanied by its own set of ethical considerations. This can best be illustrated by an extreme example — the way in which bodies were obtained in the early years of medical education in Britain.

Obtaining bodies for dissection

Historical developments

Early dissections in Britain (from the sixteenth century onwards) were of criminals executed for murder. The result of this was that dissection became recognized as a punishment, since it was something over and above execution itself. In 1752 an Act of Parliament gave judges discretion in death sentences for murder, and this was to substitute dissection for gibbeting in chains. Since gibbeting was regarded as a grim fate, dissection became recognized as being as bad, if not worse. The intention of both was to deny burial to the wrongdoer. A further punitive element of dissection is that it did something to the body *beyond* that already inflicted on the scaffold.

This means of acquiring bodies provided relatively few of them, and so the beginning of the eighteenth century saw the emergence of another means, namely, grave robbing. The earliest grave robbers were surgeon-anatomists or their pupils, and by the 1720s the stealing of bodies from London graveyards had become commonplace. Bodies stolen in this way, the so-called resurrected corpses, came from a breadth of society but were predominantly those of the poor. There was often a close liaison between the surgeon-anatomists (or medical schools) and the bodysnatchers (resurrectionists). The latter provided several thousand bodies annually, supplying the overall needs of the medical schools (Richardson, 1988).

As one might expect, this method of obtaining bodies caused great concern in some quarters. For instance, the *Lancet* in an editorial in 1832 stated: 'It is disgusting to talk of anatomy as a science, whilst it is cultivated by means of practices which would disgrace a nation of cannibals' (*Lancet*, 1832). The need to stop the resurrectionists led to the first Anatomy Bill in 1829, recommending the use of hospital patients (who were deemed to have given consent to the dissection of their bodies by the simple act of applying for treatment). However, dissection was to be limited to those with no relatives to bury them, or whose relatives were too poor to do so. Consequently, the poor were classed alongside the worst criminals as potential subjects for dissection. It was this aspect of the Bill that led to its rejection by the House of Lords.

The infamous Burke and Hare murders in Edinburgh, and similar ones by Bishop and Williams in London, proved of crucial significance to the history of anatomy in Britain. Ruth Richardson comments: 'That a vocation which professed "no object but that of conferring benefit on others" in healing the sick and the saving of human life should have been responsible for the commission of so many premeditated murders, was seen as an unspeakable paradox.' It appears that the deaths in Edinburgh were actually commissioned by the proprietor of an Edinburgh medical school, and yet he was never investigated in connection with the Burke and Hare murders. This proprietor considered that the receipt of murdered bodies was a 'mere misfortune', which would almost certainly have occurred to anybody else in his situation.

Around 1830, four options for obtaining bodies were considered and, although there had been a steady stream of bequests between 1828 and 1831, this option was not taken seriously and the 1832 Act reflected the medical opinion that the most uncontroversial source would be the use of 'unclaimed bodies'. This made poverty the sole criterion for dissection, since the Bill abolished the use of dissection as a punishment for murder.

The major contrast between the 1832 Bill and the unsuccessful one of 1829 was deletion of any references to hospitals and workhouses.

The social status of the proposed subjects of dissection had been deleted, although the intentions of the Bill remained exactly as before. As a result, in the 100 years after the Anatomy Act was passed in 1832, 57,000 bodies were dissected in the London anatomy schools. Less than 0.5 per cent came from anywhere other than institutions housing the poor, either workhouses or asylums. In the early years of this century, as the workhouses provided fewer bodies, asylums provided comparatively more.

In Britain, the number of bequests remained extremely low until the 1940s, and not until the 1960s did this source account for 70 per cent. The reasons for this dramatic change in attitude have not been adequately investigated, although they probably include changes in the social meaning of the corpse paralleling as they do a rise in the popularity of cremation, growing disbelief in the spiritual significance of the corpse, a growing awareness of the role and value of scientific medicine, and changing attitudes towards poverty.

The New Zealand experience

Developments in New Zealand have, inevitably, been much shorter, stemming as they do from the beginnings of the University of Otago Medical School in 1875. From 1876 to 1886 practically all the bodies came from Dunedin Public Hospital, after which it served only a minor role until recent times. By 1900 the Benevolent Institution (the poor house) had become the major source of supply, and this continued through to the early 1920s (Jones and Fennell, 1991). In the early 1900s, a third source of bodies appeared on the scene, namely, the mental hospitals. One in particular, Seacliff Mental Hospital, proved a prolific source of bodies, especially from 1916 to 1930. The supply from this hospital was augmented by that from other mental hospitals from around 1920 to the late 1950s.

The first record of a bequest is in 1943, but these only became more frequent during the 1950s, and did not become the major means of supply until the early 1960s and thereafter. Unclaimed bodies continued to be sent from mental hospitals through to the late 1950s. In short, the unclaimed poor provided practically the entire supply of bodies from 1889 to 1902, and from then until 1915 an average of 50 per cent. When this supply began to dry up, the potential hiatus was readily filled by the mental hospitals, so much so that it was the outcasts of society languishing in mental hospitals that provided most bodies in the first half of this century.

Society's (and the medical profession's) willingness to utilize bodies in the absence of informed consent prior to death on the part of the 'donors' has been a reflection of society's (and the medical profession's) attitudes towards the poor and the mentally ill. In this regard, the history of anatomy in New Zealand has been characterized by a consensus in which the educational value of dissection and possible future medical benefits stemming from dissection have been regarded as outweighing the autonomy of the disadvantaged within society. In this New Zealand was not alone. Moreover, it is a situation that has not applied for the past thirty years in this country (although it still applies in some countries). For us it is, therefore, a matter chiefly of historical interest, and yet the ethical considerations that apply here are relevant in many other contexts in which human material is used.

New Zealand legislation

Although there have been changes in legislation in New Zealand over the past 120 years or so, we shall deal only with current legislation. This is the Human Tissue Act of 1964.

According to this Act, the voluntary donation of bodies is paramount. However, still present is the possibility that the person lawfully in possession of the body (medical superintendent of a hospital, mental hospital, or penal institution) may authorize the body to be used for the purposes of anatomical examination, unless the deceased person had expressed an objection to this or a surviving spouse or relative does so. A second point is that the deceased person's wishes regarding donating his or her body can be over-ridden by the objections of a surviving spouse or relative. Third, there is no reference to the length of time the remains may be kept prior to burial or cremation, and it is explicitly stated that 'any part of the body may be retained indefinitely for further study'. Emphasis is placed on avoiding unnecessary mutilation of the body, and also on carrying out the examination in 'an orderly, quiet and decent manner'.

Persons and bodies

The major stipulations in this Act (or equivalent ones in other countries) raise an important ethical query, and this is: Why do we think in these ways? Why do we stress that bodies should be treated in a 'decent' manner, and why do we emphasize the wishes of the spouse? Any answer will probably have various components.

The first component is that a person is so closely identified with his or her body, that the two become more-or-less inseparable. We recognize each other because we recognize each other's bodies, in particular, the appearance, voice, and attitudes of other people. What is more, some very important aspects of this identity continue even when the person is dead. One writer has expressed it like this: '. . . while the body retains a recognizable form, even in death, it commands the respect of identity. No longer a human presence, it still reminds us of the presence that once was utterly inseparable from it' (May, 1985).

Robert Wennberg, a philosopher, refers to this as the 'overflow principle': 'We don't treat human corpses as garbage, because the corpse is closely associated with persons: it is the remains of a physical organism that at one time supported and made possible personal life' (Wennberg, 1985).

The second component, and closely associated with this, are other people's responses to the cadaver. Those who knew the person when alive have memories of that person: what she was like, her personality, her foibles, her beliefs, her hobbies. The cadaver, therefore, has – in a sense – a whole array of built-in memories, which can never be completely separated from it. For most people, these memories lead to the feeling that a corpse should be respected. In a similar way, most people are horrified when a corpse is deliberately desecrated in some manner.

We respect the person who *was*, as we remember that person. All that remains of the person is the corpse, and yet our respect for that person and for the memory of that person leads to respect for the person's remains. There is a link that is not readily broken.

In the third place, the deceased person was, in most instances, someone's relative or someone's friend. That relative or friend is now grieving the death, and so respect for the cadaver is respect for their grief. Although it is true that this will decrease as time passes, this is not to deny the importance of the cadaver as an integral part of the grief process.

These considerations leave unanswered questions regarding precisely what can or cannot be done to cadavers in an Anatomy Department's Dissecting Room. By themselves, they provide no justification for dissection, and they provide no assistance in helping us understand why such bodies can be dismembered in ways society would not contemplate allowing on 'ordinary' cadavers. One reason, although perhaps not very convincing, is that society allows this under very stringent conditions. However, as we have already seen in looking at the history of dissection, society may tolerate unethical practices in this realm, and undoubtedly some societies still do. A far more important reason ethically is that the bodies have been donated for this purpose, by those who have made a free and informed decision prior to their death. They decided that this is what they wanted to become of their bodies after death. In other words, they have made a gift of them, freely willing their own bodies to be used in this manner for educational purposes. In doing this, they have made a gift of something more closely identified than anything else with what they are. The crucial element here is the 'gift' element, something that might be interpreted as the height of altruism (May, 1985).

Use of material from unethical experiments

The emphasis on carrying out ethical research today has to be seen against a background of some of the unethical studies conducted in previous years. Two examples will be referred to, one of grossly unethical research, and the other of culturally controversial research.

Nazi research

It is not often that histology slides used for teaching undergraduate students make headline news, and yet such was the case in the late 1980s. At that time, there were claims that tissue samples from the corpses of victims of the Nazi executions were being used for teaching purposes in German medical schools. It had long been known that corpses for medical education had been obtained from execution sites from as early as 1933, reaching a peak during the height of the Nazi era in the early 1940s. Consequently, it would have been most surprising if at least some of the tissue had not come from people killed unethically by the Nazis in concentration camps.

A related, longer-standing controversy is that of the citing of data from Nazi experiments. This allied controversy illustrates the point that scientific research has at least two ethical aspects to it: the research itself (and how it is carried out), and the data resulting from the research. Since research may be conducted in an ethical or in an unethical manner, some people argue that the results of the research may be ethically acceptable (if the research was ethical) or ethically unacceptable (if the research was unethical). There are, therefore, two related controversies over the use of Nazi-derived human material, although the ethical principle at stake is the same: it is that of moral complicity. According to this, those who use material or data obtained unethically are themselves implicated in the unethical practices. It is as if they are themselves acting unethically.

Only two responses to this are possible: either the principle is accepted and any use of the material or data is rejected, or the principle is rejected and any of the material or data considered of scientific merit is used as any ethically-derived material or data would be used. These two mutually exclusive responses can be better appreciated by considering the arguments in a little more detail.

The first reason for refusing to use the material or data stems from respect shown for those killed under totally unethical circumstances. It is argued that respect is most clearly demonstrated by cremating any remains still extant, and by refusing to use them or any Nazi-derived data for any scientific or clinical purposes today. Only in this way can a nation's guilt be obviated.

A second reason is that doing so implicates us today in Nazi crimes. By using the material, we become one with the perpetrators of the original crimes, since our motives today cannot be isolated from the manner in which the material was obtained. Even to cite unethical work is to validate it, and to demonstrate that there is a continuing thread connecting respectable research today to ethically abhorrent work in the Nazi era (Max, 1989). This is the essence of the moral complicity argument.

A third reason for refusing to use the material or data is that the attitudes of the medical profession that allowed so many physicians to participate in Nazi policy-making and exterminating practice are not far removed from the attitudes of some more recent physicians. All unethical attitudes need to be explored and rejected, and a radical transformation of attitudes is only possible by refusing to have anything to do with work that has emanated from unethical behaviour.

The opposite stance, a willingness to use Nazi-based material or data, is based on a perceived ability to separate the evil of the original act from the good intentions of any contemporary work. This rejects the notion of moral complicity.

The first argument here is that, whatever we may think of them, the material and data (obtained unethically) exist. If the data are valid, they cannot be invalidated, no matter how objectionable we may find the unethical behaviour used to obtain them. Raw data obtained unethically are no different from raw data obtained ethically. In fact, since such data are unobtainable using today's much more rigorous ethical standards, they are of especial significance. However, there is a major proviso, and this is that the data are valid scientifically. Some also argue that good may be derived from evil, provided the horror is addressed (Moe, 1984).

A second argument is that it is ethically acceptable to utilize data obtained unethically since the scientific and clinical studies carried out today, on the basis of clearly delineated and accepted ethical principles, have no link to studies carried out in the 1930s and 1940s on the basis of concepts such as that of racial hygiene. While great care is required to ensure that such concepts never again become a part of medical research, this will be achieved by an understanding of ethical principles and not by a refusal to utilize any valid data from those earlier studies. According to those who use this argument, society at large and the medical profession in particular have by now learned the crucial significance of informed consent for all medical research and treatment.

Burial of archaeological human remains

The return of skeletal remains, held in Anatomy Departments, Medical Schools, and Museums, to tribes for subsequent reburial has become a commonplace issue in recent times. For example, the University of Edinburgh was reported in early 1991 as having returned nine Tasmanian Aboriginal skulls, housed for more than a century in its Anatomy Department, to Australian government representatives. They included the skull believed to be that of the last male Tasmanian Aboriginal, William Lanney. A descendant of Lanney's, a Tasmanian lawyer, had been a leader in the campaign for the repatriation of the skulls.

The issue is that of the ownership of archaeological human remains, with some policies stipulating that skeletal remains of named individuals be returned to identifiable descendants, or that remains associated with a surviving tribe be returned to that tribe. This does not take into account the large numbers of prehistoric remains in some collections, since there is no way of associating these remains with any modern descendants.

The tension here is between scientific interest and its need/hunger for the provision of valuable clues to humanity's past, against the sacred feelings and beliefs of indigenous peoples. Some argue that human skeletal artefacts provide essential information on problems ranging from the organization of tribal societies to the origin of certain diseases such as rheumatoid arthritis. It is also argued that these remains are part of the world's heritage, and are not simply of significance to the direct ancestors of the people who happen to live in an area today. The indigenous position stresses the religious and cultural importance of respect for the remains of tribal ancestors; it may include a desire for restitution in the face of past mistreatment, and may also be part of a struggle for rights and recognition. It is sometimes argued that much of the material is not used, and that any information derived from these studies is not passed on to, or shared with, the indigenous communities themselves. Although this controversy is far removed from clinical medicine, it does raise important ethical considerations, some of which are of relevance in a broader context.

We must surely respect the beliefs and feelings of indigenous peoples since this is to respect them as human persons. Inherent within this is respect for their ancestors now dead, as long as there is a traceable line back to the remains as those of their ancestors.

A second point is that there is an ethical interest in human material because of the close association that is generally recognized between such material and a known and recognizable human person. However, this probably does not apply with anything like the same force when no link can be established with any known person or group of people. Nevertheless, it is still material of human origin that tells us something about its associations, even when these have been forgotten. Some indigenous groups also recognize it as an essential part of their history and ancestry. In other words, even ancient human material does not become nothing simply because of the loss of links with the present.

Third, there is a place for the scientific study of archaeological human remains, since this is a particular application of the more general principle that the study of human material is important and ethically acceptable. However, in this instance, no one consented to the study of these remains, since none of the direct descendants could do so. This either renders any study of archaeological human remains unethical, or consent in this instance is irrelevant. A compromise position is to seek proxy consent from present-day descendants, if such can be identified. What this leads to is an agreement between archaeologists and indigenous communities to allow a defined time for scientific study of the remains prior to reburial. It is to be hoped that such a co-operative solution is made earlier rather than later in a context of communion with and sensitivity to the concerns of any descendants.

A fourth consideration is to ask whether material resulting (in part, at least) from past mistreatment of some indigenous peoples should be studied at all. This touches on the moral complicity issues brought out far more poignantly in the previous discussion of Nazi-derived data.

Can the dead body be abused?

In this section, we move on a step from the issues considered above where living people were (or may have been) abused. To us today it seems that the abuse of living people is unethical, although, as we have just seen, there is no consensus as to how we deal with the present-day results of abuse that occurred in the past. Although there is no question that people can be treated in unethical ways, can cadavers or dead people be treated in unethical ways? This brings us back to the sorts of issues raised earlier in this chapter. Who is being treated unethically now that the person himself is dead? In what sense can a dead person, someone who is no longer with us, be abused? Is it the memory others have of that person that is being abused? Alternatively, it may be the human race that is somehow demeaned when one of their kind (even though now dead) is treated in a less-than-human way. But what is a less-than-human way? What does this mean when thinking about a dead person?

These are not easy questions, if we expect to provide clear rational answers rather than respond on the basis of intuitive feelings. Alternatively, it may be that our intuition on this matter is an important pointer to the sort of treatment we think should or should not be inflicted on the bodies of those who were once like us.

Three illustrations may help at this point.

Research on the clinically dead

In 1988 the death was reported in France of a young man, killed in a car accident, whose body had been used for a medical experiment while in a deep coma. The doctor involved had placed the patient on sabotaged medical equipment. He was attempting to determine whether the effects were the same as in a similar previous instance in which he had been involved. The doctor behind these experiments has called such patients 'almost perfect human models, who constitute intermediaries between animal and man'.

These two experiments led to storms of protest, and the doctor was suspended from his duties. In the 1985 experiment, the patient, who was brain-dead, was subjected to an experiment involving a high-speed blood transfusion into a pelvic bone. Objections to this experiment were based principally on the lack of informed consent by the patient. To some, the patient was treated as an object rather than a human subject, an attitude that exemplifies medical imperialism. To others, however, the existence of brain death allows for some experimentation on techniques of reanimation.

However, these responses do not appear to bring the matter to a close. Let us assume that informed consent for this type of experimentation had been given prior to death. Would there, then, be any ethical objections to it? What would be the difference between this experimentation and dissecting a cadaver? It is difficult to see that there is any difference, as long as there is no deception of the relatives, and as long as the nature of the experimentation is known and agreed to by an appropriate ethics committee.

Trauma research

In 1978 the Department of Transportation in California had contracted with several university laboratories to test designs for automobile air bags in actual crashes of cars at varying velocities. Since dummies had proved unsatisfactory for measuring the degree of protection for living passengers, some researchers had, with the consent of next-of-kin, substituted human cadavers. One congressman wrote to the Secretary of Transportation charging that 'the use of human cadavers for vehicle safety research violates fundamental notions of morality and human dignity, and must therefore permanently be stopped'. It was stopped, despite the Department's protest that prohibition of the use of cadavers would set back progress on safety protection for many years.

The question raised by this instance is: what is the difference between these experiments or dissection? Next-of-kin had given their consent for the experiments, and no attempt was made to carry them out in a secretive way. Hence, the objections to the studies in the previous section do not apply here. Why, then, the outcry? Was this on ethical grounds or on emotional ones?

There is no doubt that there are major differences between the airbag experiments and dissection, in that the cadavers in the former are violently smashed to bits, whereas dissection is carried out in laboratories by medical technicians or students. Dissection is analytical and scientific, whereas smashing bodies is violent and destructive. It has been suggested that the difference is a symbolic one (Feinberg, 1985). The end-result in both situations is destruction: generally far greater destruction in the case of dissection than in the case of the airbag experiments. A symbolic difference suggests that what is significant is the manner in which the destruction is brought about, with the violent form of destruction being offensive to some societies today. If this is the case, it must be regarded as a relative matter, since what societies will tolerate at any particular time is relative. After all, dissection was not tolerated by most societies just a few hundred years ago. So what we deem unacceptable today may be considered quite acceptable a few years hence.

We have to decide whether peoples' intuition in this matter is a reliable guide, since the expected safety benefit of experiments such as these has to be balanced against the offence experienced by some people.

Undoubtedly, some people are offended by dissection, but they are able to steer clear of it (unless they are medical and some other health science students). It is difficult to see why human dignity should be placed in jeopardy by destructive experiments, but not by dissection.

The age of the neomort

In a now famous article Willard Gaylin takes a scientific fiction look at what society could do with cadavers (Gaylin, 1974). In this, Gaylin imagined institutions of the future where brain-dead bodies, now euphemistically called 'neomorts', are maintained and put to various important medical uses. The bioemporiums would resemble a cross between a pharmaceutical laboratory and a hospital ward. He envisages hospital beds lined up in neat rows, each with a freshly scrubbed neomort under the clean white sheets. The neomorts will have the same recognizably human faces they had before they died, the same features, even the same complexions. Each would be a perfect natural symbol not only of humanity in general, but of the particular person who once animated the body and had their life in it.

Using such 'preparations', medical students could be taught the techniques of rectal or vaginal examination without fear of disturbing or embarrassing real patients. Experiments could be performed to test the toxicity of drugs by judging their effects on real human bodies without endangering anyone's health or life. Other neomorts could be used as experimental subjects, rather than use live animals such as dogs and mice; their advantages are that they feel no pain, and raise no ethical issues connected with animal welfare concerns. Other neomorts could serve as living organ banks or living storage receptacles for blood antigens and platelets that cannot survive freezing. From others could be harvested at regular intervals blood, bone marrow, corneas, and cartilage, as needed for transfusion or transplants by patients. Still others may be used to manufacture hormones, antitoxins, and antibodies to be marketed commercially for the prevention or cure of various medical ailments.

This may seem far-fetched, and yet some of the ethical dilemmas currently confronting the medical profession in clinical areas would be bypassed by such bioemporiums. Alarming as this scenario may be, what is important is to provide a serious ethical response based on the dignity to be ascribed to the dead and the reactions of the living to what we do to, and with, the dead. In formulating a response to this scenario, the considerations discussed in the previous sections are all relevant, especially those concerning the prior consent of the people concerned and their relatives. Consent may also be required of those making use of such emporiums, since it is ethically important to the people who may benefit from them that they approve of the source of the material. If they are horrified by where it has come from, or simply have reservations about it, their own autonomy requires the freedom to decline to participate in such a venture.

Organ transplants

It is not such a big jump from harvesting the dead to harvesting the living as we might think. So, in the final section of this chapter, we shall turn our attention to organ transplants.

The purchase of kidneys from living donors, for transplantation into the purchasing recipients, appears to be almost commonplace in some countries. In most instances, the sellers are poor and healthy, whereas the purchasers are rich and unhealthy. The reaction of many public figures to this trade in human kidneys has been one of moral outrage, the abhorrence appearing to stem principally from the notion that it is unethical to sell parts of the human body for money.

There has been widespread acceptance that relatives may donate a kidney for altruistic reasons. They are volunteers, and may well consider it a privilege to do this for a loved one – perhaps a brother or sister, husband or wife, or a son or daughter. Many, however, would not restrict such donation to a relative, as long as donors are made fully aware of the short- and long-term hazards of the procedure and that they are freely and voluntarily giving their fully informed consent to the donation. There appear to be no ethical reasons against this, and perhaps the altruism and risk-taking implicit within it are to be encouraged.

But what about selling organs? It is difficult to see why organ donation for money is inherently wrong, especially if the money is to be used to buy education or health care for a close relative. In this case it could, once again, be an example of altruism, the motives being ones of concern and care for others. In terms of a market-place philosophy, the selling of organs may serve to re-circulate cash from the haves to the have-nots.

However, some are far from convinced by arguments of this kind and have compared the selling of kidneys to prostitution. But, as with prostitution, it is difficult to identify the guilty party. Is it the donor who sells part of her body in a once-only deal, or is it the purchaser who pays what she must for what she cannot live without? Alternatively, is it the broker who makes possible the exchange, or is it the transplant surgeon desperate to help her patient? These are not easy ethical questions, especially when framed in a world characterized by frightening inequality in wealth and in access to health care, and also when there is major failure to harvest all potential cadaveric organs.

The one factor in this debate that is ethically unacceptable is the factor of exploitation. This is implicit within a market-place situation, and yet once again the question is: who is exploiting whom? There may be emotional exploitation of a reluctant donor by family members, financial exploitation of a reluctant donor by relatives or a broker, or various forms of exploitation by the medical profession and intermediaries. These are dangers inherent within any form of brokerage for profit, especially where the financial stakes are high. Not surprisingly, therefore, any financial deals for organs almost inevitably mean that it is money rather than medical need that determines which patients receive kidneys. While it may be possible to avoid this, it would be horrendously difficult to administer. Consequently, whatever procedures are permitted in this area need to be carried out under stringent guidelines designed to protect living donors from all forms of exploitation.

The inadequate supply of donor kidneys from freshly deceased people could be rectified by a more efficient harvesting of kidneys, by publicity, and possibly by legislation in favour of a 'required request' law or by an opting-out rather than an opting-in system for donations from cadavers. This still leaves another consideration, and this is that with the greater use of seat belts, crash helmets, and tougher drink driving laws there may be a decrease in the number of donor victims and therefore a decrease in the potential supply of 'brain-dead' patients. The result could be an even greater pressure on living donors as a source of kidneys.

This highlights the tension implicit within any use of human organs for transplantation – between the 'good' of the transplantation and the 'evil' of the source of the organs. This applies whether the organs come from dead or living donors. The ethical issues vary between the two groups, the emphasis in the former being on the tragedy resulting in the death, and in the latter on the risks attached to the donation procedure. The nature of the necessary informed consent also differs in the two cases, although there is an element of moral complicity in both situations.

Another issue of relevance to the harvesting of organs from a cadaver involves our concept of the totality of the body. It may be acceptable to remove the kidneys, say, from a cadaver, but what about the liver, heart, lungs, and eyes as well? In other words, does the wholesale removal of organs in some sense desecrate the body? Do we end up with little more than an empty shell, as opposed to a relatively intact body? To some relatives George, even though dead, may still be George without his kidneys, but perhaps they regard him as less-than-George when a large array of his organs has been removed. This is a response which needs to be noted. One very practical concern is the right course of action where relatives disagree with the stated wishes of the deceased. If we regard transplantation as an ethically commendable thing, then we need to think carefully about the current tendency to respect the wishes of surviving relatives. We do not regard their wishes as paramount in the resolution of the general affairs of the deceased, so it is difficult to argue that they should be so regarded in respect of organ donation. It would seem, therefore, that given an explicit gifting by a patient, the relatives should not be allowed to veto an organ donation.

Besides these specific ethical issues, more general issues are also raised by organ transplants, both from cadavers and living donors. For instance, on someone's death should they be available automatically for any surgical team which can make good use of them, or should they only be made available if the deceased has expressly stated this during his life, or if the next-of-kin have given permission?

Many pragmatic arguments can be used in favour of their free availability. For instance, there is a desperate need of kidneys and hearts for transplantation purposes. Should society move in this direction then, and state that organs can be obtained from cadavers as long as there have been no written statements expressly forbidding this during life? In other words, people would have to contract out of donating their organs at death, as opposed to the present situation whereby they have to contract in and actively express a wish that their organs are used in this way.

Whatever conclusions we come to should take into account the points made previously about cadavers in general. Of these, a crucial point is the importance of the 'gift' element in organ transplantation. This is of especial significance when organs are transplanted from a dead person. In this case, the person prior to death has decided to make a gift of parts of her own body to someone else, parts she knows will no longer be of any value to her after her death. Alternatively, the parents or spouse may be faced with the same decision on behalf of someone close to them after what was probably a tragic and untimely death. This is one way in which some good can be extracted from a tragedy. Of course, this doesn't have to involve the 'gifting' of an organ to someone else; the law could state that organs are removed automatically in the absence of a previous clear directive from the deceased to the contrary. However, it is the gift element, with its overtones of altruism, that are of especial importance morally.

Chapter 4

Issues before birth

Introduction

The ethical issues raised in the previous chapter revolve around society's view of the human body after birth. Complex as some of those issues are, they are grounded in a strong consensus that the human body is to be treated with respect and that human life is to be protected under all normal circumstances. However, when we turn to life before birth — to embryos and foetuses — a similar consensus does not hold. To many people it is not self-evident that embryonic and foetal life is to be given the same degree of protection as that given human life after birth. Besides this, other considerations, such as the autonomy of the mother, are also regarded as of major ethical significance.

The difficulty is that the status ascribed to human embryos and foetuses is far from easy to determine, and different people arrive at different conclusions. What is more, this status is arrived at on both biological and moral grounds, and neither provides definitive guidance. We shall look first at the biological component.

Biological definitions

Embryo and foetus

The term 'embryo' is traditionally used to refer to the human conceptus from fertilization until eight weeks gestation, although in recent ethical writings it is sometimes confined to the period up to implantation at two weeks gestation. This pre-implantation phase is also known as the 'pre-embryo' stage of development. While the precise terms used are somewhat arbitrary, any deviation from the traditional embryo-foetus distinction at eight weeks gestation should be undertaken only with care.

The foetal period is further subdivided into previable and viable periods. The term 'previable' refers to a foetus showing signs of life but not having the capacity to survive after separation from the mother. A foetus is generally considered to be previable when under twenty weeks gestation and weighing less than 400 grams (although these figures are relative and vary from one country to another). The term 'viable' is used of a foetus having the capacity to survive and sustain independent existence.

Fertilization

Fertilization is the fusion of a sperm and an ovum. This is achieved by penetration of the outer layers of the ovum (corona radiata and zona pellucida) by the sperm, which becomes engulfed within the cytoplasm of the ovum. These processes induce the ovum to complete its maturation, one aspect of which is the joining of the male and female pronuclei. When this is completed, the fertilized ovum is known as a *zygote*. The process of fertilization takes up to twenty-four hours to be completed, and usually takes place in the uterine tube.

Once this process has occurred, the ovum becomes active and the genetic individuality of the embryo is established by the combination of genes from each of the parents. The resulting one-celled embryo, or zygote, is still capable of splitting to form two individuals. This twinning potential remains for as long as two weeks after fertilization.

The first cell divisions of the fertilized ovum produce a cluster of equivalent cells (blastomeres), which are not integrated at this stage into a multicellular organism. This non-integrated state persists for a few days after fertilization. It has been demonstrated in mouse embryos that one or more cells can be removed from an early embryo during this period without affecting the outcome of development — a complete mouse is born. A few more days of development pass before the cells which will give rise to the embryo proper can be distinguished from the cells which will form the placenta.

The first blastomeres appear within thirty hours of fertilization, while by three days a ball (morula) of sixteen or so cells is formed. The morula enters the uterus shortly after this. It lies free in the uterine lumen for one or two days, by which time it consists of between fifty and sixty cells. During this time a fluid-filled cavity gradually develops within the morula; when this is established the whole structure is known as a blastocyst. Some of the cells form a structure that, later on, will form part of the placenta.

At about six days the blastocyst adheres to the wall of the uterus, following which some of its outer cells begin to invade the uterine wall. This is the beginning of implantation. Two or three days later the amniotic cavity makes its first appearance. By twelve to fourteen days implantation is complete, and a primitive placental circulation has developed. At this time the embryo is still a flat two-layered disc, although the first indication of the future head end of the embryo appears at about this time. The primitive streak develops as a midline thickening at fifteen to sixteen days, after which early features of the nervous system make their appearance.

Personhood of the embryo and foetus

The difficulties associated with deciding when 'life' begins biologically, are more than matched by the difficulties in determining when persons come into existence. Of course, the two issues are not quite this separate in real life, since there are large areas of overlap between the biological and the philosophical.

> Imagine the following scene. Cheryl has just become aware that she is pregnant, since she has missed two periods and she has had the pregnancy confirmed. An embryo has been in existence for about six weeks. There is no doubt there is new biological life within Cheryl; this will either keep on developing, or something will go wrong and she will miscarry. Either way, she will be aware of it. Cheryl is delighted at being pregnant, and she refers to this embryo as her child. What does she mean by this term? She knows what children are like, of course; her sister has a three-year-old. But is her six-week-old embryo a child in the same way as the three-year-old is a child? It will probably become a child, but is it one now?
>
> Let's now consider an alternative possibility. Cheryl never intended to become pregnant, and now wants to have an abortion. For her, the embryo is nothing like a child; it's a nuisance since she has other plans for the next two years and these don't include having a child. An abortion presents her with no moral difficulties, since for her a six-week-old embryo is nothing special in human terms.
>
> A third possibility sees Cheryl wanting her pregnancy to continue. However, she has no desire to refer to the embryo within her as a child. She hopes everything will continue satisfactorily, but she is unable at this early stage to feel that she is carrying a complete new human being. If anything goes wrong, she will probably be upset, but she will not actually consider she has lost a child.

These three scenes correspond to the three major viewpoints on the moral status of prenatal human life: embryos/foetuses are persons, they are non-persons, or they are potential persons. We shall now look at each of these in turn.

Foetuses are persons

According to this stance, the embryo is to be regarded (and therefore treated) as a human person from the time of fertilization. Some argue that, since it is impossible to prove that personhood begins later than fertilization, moral prudence should err on the conservative side and conclude that personhood probably begins at fertilization. Whatever the precise formulation, the outcome is the same: from fertilization the embryo is to be treated in the same way we would treat a mature human person (McCormick, 1981).

According to this viewpoint, the process of embryonic development is nothing less than the development of a person. There is no stage in human existence when we are not persons (Iglesias, 1984). A corollary of this is that embryos and foetuses are to be accorded absolute respect and are to be treated as inviolable. Underlying these conclusions is one idea of potentiality: whatever we now are, was present in potential form in the embryos from which we developed. Since we now have self-consciousness, the potential for self-consciousness must be present in all embryos. Therefore, it is argued, all embryos possess personal life, and are actual persons with considerable potential.

The question, however, is whether the capacity of *a* to develop into A makes *a* exactly the same as A. Quite obviously, the ability of an acorn to develop into an oak tree does not convert the acorn into an oak tree. Conversely, to destroy an acorn is not the same as destroying an oak tree. A three-day-old embryo is not the same as a thirty-year-old human adult. Although the potential is undoubtedly there, the actual adult is far from realization in a three-day-old embryo.

In no other area of life do we equate the potential with the actual. For instance, a student commencing a course of study has the potential to pass the final examinations, and this potential may ultimately be realized when the examinations are passed. In order to accomplish this, however, a great deal of teaching and learning is required, and it is these alone that convert the potential for success into actual success. Along the way, however, the student is changed by the learning, so that the student who passes the examination is *different* from the student who turned up at the first class with a potential for passing the examination (Jones, 1987).

To argue like this does not convert an embryo into a 'nothing', any more than the student in the above analogy is regarded as a 'failed' student, or is excluded from further study on the grounds that he has not as yet passed the final examinations. This, however, is to jump ahead of ourselves.

Foetuses are non-persons

One argument in favour of the non-personhood of embryos and foetuses stems from the generally-held viewpoint that we do not consider it wrong to destroy either the ovum or sperm before they have united. From this, some argue that we are not morally obliged to preserve the life of the embryo. If this is so, the embryo may be regarded as a thing, rather than as a person, until that point in development when some brain function can be detected (Singer and Wells, 1984).

According to this viewpoint, the first few weeks of gestation have no moral significance. The complete lack of any personhood (either actual or potential) places no moral obligations on the human community. The embryo, as a non-sentient being, has no moral rights. The point at which this situation changes is open to debate. Considerable emphasis is placed by some writers on the acquisition by the embryo or foetus of consciousness, or at least a potential for consciousness. This, in turn, depends on some minimum degree of nervous system development. The emphasis here is on the acquisition of sentience, that is, the ability to feel pleasure or pain. This, it is argued, signifies that an embryo or foetus has sufficient moral status to make it wrong to do certain things to it, for example, to inflict unnecessary pain upon it.

If this argument is accepted, it has to be asked at what stage of brain development consciousness is able to be manifested. From a neurobiological angle this is a difficult, if not impossible, task; and yet, it is an essential one if the embryo or foetus from this point onwards is to be the bearer of moral rights. Stages from six weeks of gestation all the way through to twenty-eight weeks of gestation have been quoted as the beginning of a 'brain', or, using different terminology, as the earliest indication of consciousness. Whatever one makes of these widely divergent appraisals, they cast doubt on the advisability of using any of these possibilities as the definitive beginning-point of personhood (Jones, 1989).

An alternative case for the non-personhood of the embryo and foetus is based on drawing a distinction between *being a human being* in the biological sense and *being a person* in the moral sense. When this is done, it can readily be concluded that not all human beings are persons.

This, in turn, raises the inevitable question of whether or not the foetus is a person. If we expect of a person properties such as being able to recall past states, envisage a future for itself, and having personality traits that do not alter too drastically over short periods of time, foetuses are not persons. Similarly, however, neither are young infants, adults in a vegetative state, or adults with severe dementia, persons. On the other hand, the adult members of some animal species, such as some primates and dolphins, may be persons.

Michael Tooley (1983) who has enunciated this approach very clearly, concedes that human foetuses and neonates are potential persons.

However, he also argues that potential personhood only allows us to confer a right to life (for foetuses and infants), if we also accept the principle that it is wrong to refrain from producing additional persons. If one assumes that we are under no obligation to produce children (that is, contraception is acceptable), Tooley concludes that the killing of a foetus (a potential person) is no worse than using contraceptives.

A problem with this approach is what one commentator has described as the 'moral obligation to nurture' (Sommers, 1985). It fails to take account of the commitments humans have to the welfare and survival of infants and also, to varying extents, of foetuses. The human family has obligations, since the newborn is totally dependent on the voluntary acts of responsible moral agents committed to its care. Apart from such interactions, neither foetuses nor the newborn would survive. In other words, neurological and behavioural factors alone are not sufficient to tell us how we should act towards foetuses and infants (and also seriously impaired adults), since they fail to take account of the commitments that are so essential to life together within the human community. Even inadequate ratings on a biological scale of values have to be viewed within this social context, since the notion of personhood incorporates social as well as intellectual factors. What they attest is that, even when the neurological and behavioural features of the foetus or newborn are inadequate on a biological scale of values, our commitment to love and care for one of our own is basic to what we are as humans living in community.

Foetuses are potential persons

A third perspective occupies a place somewhere between these two. It views the foetus as a being with the potential for full personhood. According to this perspective, in the normal course of its development, the foetus (as a potential person) will acquire a person's claim to life, although even early on in its development it already has some claim to life (Langerak, 1979). In terms of this principle, a human foetus is a potential person, as opposed to an actual person (a normal adult human being), a being with a capacity for personhood (a temporarily unconscious person), a possible person (a human sperm or ovum), or a future person (a person in a future generation). In practical terms, potential persons, such as foetuses, have some claim to life, whereas possible persons have no such claim.

Emphasis on this sort of potential takes seriously the continuum of biological development, and does not draw an arbitrary line to denote the acquisition of personhood. At all stages of development the foetus is on its way to full personhood and, if everything proceeds normally, it will one day attain full personhood in its own right.

According to this viewpoint, there is no point in development, no matter how early on, when the embryo or foetus doesn't display some elements of personhood — no matter how rudimentary. The potential is there, and it is because of this that both the embryo and foetus have a claim to life and respect. This claim, however, becomes stronger as foetal development proceeds, so that by some time during the third trimester the claim is so strong that the consequences of killing a foetus are the same as those of killing an actual person — whether child or adult. Consequently, the foetus in the last trimester will, when necessary, be treated as a 'patient'. This mirrors most people's responses in ordinary life, where we recognize a difference between the accidental loss of an embryo or early foetus and the birth of a stillborn child. Both entail the death of human life, and yet under most circumstances the loss of a life which 'almost-made-it' is felt much more acutely than that of a life which had 'hardly-begun-to-develop'.

As with all intermediate positions, the potential person position satisfies neither extreme. It is seen as being too liberal by those advocating a 'foetus is a person' viewpoint, and too conservative by the 'foetus is not a person' school. Not only this, but the 'potential person' stance is itself open to varying interpretations. Nevertheless, its gradualist emphasis strikes a chord with many, on biological, philosophical, intuitive, and pragmatic grounds. It helps many through the maze of problems in the difficult prenatal and neonatal areas, and constitutes a helpful ethical basis for tackling specific ethical issues in this present chapter.

Research on foetuses and embryos

Foetal research

Over recent years three types of research have been carried out on foetuses: those performed in the uterus prior to abortion or normal delivery; those performed in the uterus during an abortion; and those performed outside the uterus following an abortion, and therefore following separation from the mother.

The first type of research includes many non-invasive therapeutic procedures, with the research being an offshoot of diagnostic or therapeutic procedures, such as studies of foetal behaviour in response to sound. However, other studies are different: for example, live rubella

(German measles) vaccine has been administered to mothers more than a week prior to induced abortion, in an attempt to discover whether accidental administration of this vaccine during pregnancy has any effect on the foetus. Other research has been carried out to investigate the transfer of substances, such as radio-isotopes, across the placenta, a few hours before abortion, with the aborted foetus subsequently being examined for traces of the substance in question.

In the second type of study, radioactive isotopes have been injected into the umbilical vein of the foetus during abortion by hysterotomy, with the mother being examined for the presence of radioactivity. The aim of such experiments is to discover whether compounds are transported across the placenta from the foetal to the maternal side.

In the third type of study, aborted foetuses have been examined following separation from the mother. Since aborted foetuses may continue to live following abortion by hysterotomy or hysterectomy, some aspects of foetal physiology can be investigated. One example in the literature has been the study of the circulatory system in the uterus and placenta by outlining the blood vessels by the injection of a barium sulphate solution. Another investigation involved the removal of foetal organs and tissues from still-living foetuses immediately following abortion. The aim of studies such as these was to investigate the synthesis of certain substances in the liver and brain of the foetus.

Following the publication of studies like these, many people raised practical and ethical objections to them. As a result, in various countries committees were set up in the 1970s and early 1980s (Reports, 1972). These concluded that experimentation on live previable foetuses was permissible within certain limits. The rationale was that important biomedical knowledge, that could not be obtained by alternative means, could be obtained using such approaches. This included knowledge about the transfer of substances across the placenta, and the reaction of foetuses to drugs.

All published guidelines build various safeguards into their provisions. In regard to experiments carried out on the foetus *in anticipation of an abortion*, minimal or no risk should be imposed on the foetus by the research. This is because the foetus may subsequently be born alive, or the woman may change her mind regarding the abortion. For experiments on the previable foetus *during the abortion procedure* or *following an abortion*, even potentially harmful research is allowed. The conditions are that the method of abortion should destroy the foetus before its complete separation from the mother, the foetus should be less than twenty weeks gestational age, the research should not lead to any alterations in the abortion procedure, and the duration of life of the foetus should not be affected by the experimental manipulations.

Research is also feasible on the dead foetus outside the uterus, and on the viable foetus either inside or outside the uterus. Most agree that a dead foetus should be treated in the same manner as any dead human individual. In this instance, consent must have been given by the mother. In the case of a viable foetus after delivery, even after an abortion, most would argue that the ethical obligation is to sustain its life and that it is unethical to experiment on it in any way that would jeopardize its life.

These guidelines appear to be saying that, once the death of the foetus is inevitable, at the time of the abortion or subsequent to it, it can be exposed to risk. The argument appears to be that, since the previable foetus is doomed, any harm resulting from the experimentation is of little consequence compared with the much greater harm caused by the abortion. Hence, if abortion is allowable, so is research on the foetus.

In general, the various guidelines adopt an intermediate position on the status of the foetus. They are not based on the view that the human foetus should be accorded the status of a person from the earliest stages of development, thereby debarring any experimentation on it. Neither do they view the foetus as a non-personal organism, since they proscribe causing harm to the living previable foetus. This intermediate position raises a number of general queries, which are of help in focusing attention on dilemmas inherent in foetal research. The fact that the foetuses are doomed (they are about to be aborted) plays a crucial role in all aspects of experimentation on live previable foetuses. The argument appears to be that, since these foetuses will never be able to realize their potential as fully-developed persons, it is legitimate to use them for the good of medical science, and therefore for the good of other foetuses that will realize that potential. However, if this position is accepted, we need to ask whether children and adults who are also doomed (for whatever reason) can be used for the good of medical science. Should experimentation on them be justified for equivalent reasons? If we answer these questions in the negative, because of major differences in the status of prenatal and postnatal human life, we have to determine the ethical nature of these differences.

Another issue concerns the nature of the parental consent that allows experimentation to be performed on live previable foetuses. This is generally based on the notion of the consent required to experiment on children, that is, the consent of the mother or parents. However, there is a difference between the nature of the consent in two instances. With children, the consent is for research on a being for whom one expects to shoulder reponsibility in the future. With previable foetuses, however, the consent refers to a being for whom the parents will not have to bear any responsibility in the future. In addition, since the parents have consented to abortion, they hardly have the best interests of the *foetus* at heart (except perhaps when the abortion is on the grounds of severe foetal abnormality). It is unlikely, therefore, that any consent they give for non-therapeutic research on the foetus will have the same meaning as consent for similar research on a child whom they want to live and for whom they hope to care.

Embryo research

Embryo research, like foetal research, has become a reality because of prior human intervention in the reproductive process. The intervention in the case of foetal research is abortion; in the case of embryo research it is *in vitro fertilization* (IVF) and the production of spare embryos. In neither case, however, does the research follow inevitably from the other procedure, although without the other procedure there could be no research of the types we are envisaging.

The debate, therefore, revolves not around the embryo *per se* but around the pre-implantation embryo outside the human body, an embryo produced by technical means. In looking at embryo research, we are concerned with embryos produced by IVF but not transferred to a woman's uterus for subsequent development.

Embryos such as these can be produced in a number of ways. They may be: superfluous to the needs of a couple in a clinical IVF programme ('spare' embryos); produced in the laboratory (using donated ovum and sperm) with the sole intention of employing them in a research programme; or the by-product of another research programme aimed at studying, for example, the fertilizing capacity of human ova or sperm.

The research imperative stems from the potential value of these pre-implantation human embryos in the furtherance of a wide range of scientific and clinical objectives (Royal Society, 1990). The most important research areas are expected to be as follows.

The treatment of infertility through IVF

The argument here is that years of research on human embryological material were needed to develop IVF to its present state of clinical practice. However, the success rate is still low and so several fertilized eggs are generally replaced in the mother's uterus in order to ensure a reasonable chance that a child will be born. A consequence of this practice is a high incidence of multiple births, with all the problems these entail for both the babies themselves and their mothers. Hence, further research is needed to improve the viability of cultured and frozen fertilized eggs (ova) before there is any prospect that their replacement in the uterus one at a time will become a practical alternative. However, if this does become feasible one day, it will signify a major advance, since it will dispense with the hormonal treatment of the mother that is currently required to obtain sufficient eggs for IVF procedures.

Preventing genetic disease

Currently, the only way of preventing the transmission of genetic disease is to test foetuses at eight to sixteen weeks gestation, and to abort those that are affected. Research on human embryos offers the prospect of testing them or developing eggs at an early stage to identify those that will be affected by, or carry, serious genetic diseases, such as Duchenne muscular dystrophy or cystic fibrosis, and of replacing in the uterus only those found to be free of such defective genes. Research on diagnosing genetic diseases between two and five days after fertilization has already made considerable advances but, it is argued, additional work is required to take this further. This requires the study of individual cells removed from developing embryos. While such work can be carried out on mouse embryos, it is essential to ascertain that the removal of cells from the fertilized *human* egg will not adversely affect its subsequent development, before such pre-implantation diagnosis can be applied clinically.

Improving contraception

Any major progress in developing simple and reliable methods of contraception depends on improved understanding of fundamental aspects of human embryology. This can only come from the study of human embryos themselves.

Research conducted on human embryos is generally carried out using guidelines. While these may differ from one country to another, they tend to have much in common. For instance, research should be scientifically valid and clinically relevant, the objectives could not be obtained by research on animals alone, consent of the donors must always be obtained, consent of a local ethical committee must always be obtained, certain lines of work (e.g. genetic modification) should be prohibited, no fertilized egg which has been experimented upon should be replaced in the uterus, and no fertilized egg should be grown for more than fourteen days *in vitro*.

The possibility of research on embryos is, not surprisingly, proving extremely contentious (Walters, 1979). For some, the human status of these embryos precludes their use in research under any circumstances. For others, the potential medical and scientific benefits for ameliorating mental and physical suffering are so great that they justify unlimited research using human embryos. These responses mirror two of the positions on foetuses (as persons, and as non-persons) discussed previously.

For those in the first group, research is morally wrong because the embryos, no matter how young and undeveloped, are human, with a potential for full human personhood. To some in this group, the human embryo (both pre- and post-implantation) should be accorded the same status as a child or adult. This moral principle is considered to outweigh any of the possible medical benefits of the research. For those in the second group, it is morally wrong not to do everything possible to alleviate human suffering, whether this is the suffering of infertility or of a genetic or chromosomal disorder, such as Down's syndrome.

Those in the first group disapprove of any research at all on the human embryo. It is forbidden territory. Those in the second group allow research, although accept an upper limit on the age at which embryos can be used for research purposes. The basis for an upper age limit is generally the appearance of neurological structures or characteristics that may signify the earliest appearance of sentience. Since the human embryo may be regarded as little more than a useful tool in the furtherance of scientific and medical advance, research procedures should not be restricted any more than is necessary. Human embryos may also be produced specifically for experimental studies.

Between these two extremes there is a medley of intermediate positions. Most reports issued by governmental and medical bodies have adopted an intermediate position (Report of Committee of Inquiry into Human Fertilisation and Embryology, 1984), although with a clear bias towards the legitimacy of some research on human embryos. When this is the case, a fourteen-day time limit on research is generally invoked. The reason for this limit is that the primitive streak, which forms at about fifteen days after fertilization, marks the beginning of individual development of the embryo.

Before drawing out some principles on the use of embryos in research, there is one consideration that deserves a more detailed discussion, and this is the notion of therapeutic and non-therapeutic research in relation to embryo experimentation. Research is generally subdivided into three categories.

In the first category, information may be relevant to the *individual embryo* on which the research is being conducted. A futuristic example is gene therapy, where the intended result is that that embryo will be given an opportunity to develop into a mature individual with an improved genetic constitution. This is *therapeutic research* in its simplest form, although there are probably no examples of this available at present.

A second possibility is that the information may be relevant to *embryos in general*, as in research aimed at decreasing the incidence of, or treating, infertility. This may involve the selection of a normal embryo from among a few embryos, in order that just one embryo will be allowed to develop to term. Alternatively, it may require the sacrifice of many present embryos so that embryos in future will benefit. The question here is whether this is therapeutic or non-therapeutic research. Reference to research on adults suggests that it is non-therapeutic, since it is not aimed at benefiting the individual on which the research is being conducted. However, we have to ask whether it is legitimate to move from a principle worked out with adult patients to one involving four-, eight-, or sixteen-cell embryos. This is an important question since only between one and five per cent of IVF embryos will give rise to living human beings, and thirty to forty per cent of naturally fertilized embryos within a woman's uterus will do the same.

A third category includes research of potential *benefit to non-embryos*, that is, to *medicine in general*. In this case, the work on embryos may be of value in the transplantation of organs or tissues, or in understanding the growth of carcinoma cells. This is clearly a *non-therapeutic* type of research since it makes use of particular embryos in order to provide information of general medical usefulness.

What does this mean in practice? Of the fifty-three research projects approved in Britain in 1989, forty-one were devoted to discovering why IVF often fails and to ways of improving the treatment of infertility, eleven were concerned with the diagnosis of genetic defects before implantation, and one involved an improved method of contraception. In other words, practically all the projects fell into the second category of research: that which is of potential benefit to embryos in general. They cannot, by definition, benefit present embryos because of the inadequacy of the techniques, but their goal is to benefit embryos in future.

The following principles are relevant to any decisions on embryo research.

First, gametes before fertilization are of lesser ethical concern than are their postfertilization products. Consequently, unfertilized eggs are not accorded comparable worth to human embryos at any postfertilization stage.

Second, embryos and foetuses deserve special respect since they are the forebears of individual humans like ourselves. This is not a universally-held principle, since the status of IVF embryos outside the uterus may differ from that of embryos fertilized naturally and existing within a woman's uterus. Another act, that of transferring them to a woman's uterus, is required. By contrast, embryos within a woman's uterus do possess this potential. This leads some to argue that IVF embryos merit no special protection. However, most consider that they do merit special protection but that this is a limited form of protection allowing research under stringent conditions. This is the most generally accepted position, although still others contend that IVF embryos merit absolute protection necessitating their placement in a woman's uterus to provide them with this potential.

Third, the embryos used for research purposes should be those that are superfluous to the needs of clinical IVF procedures. This, again, is not a generally accepted principle, but it emphasizes that the source of embryos to be used in research programmes may be of ethical significance. The deliberate production of human embryos for use in research programmes has no parallel in any other medical research. It sets out to produce organisms with the potential for full human life but which are used only as objects and never as ends in themselves. In this case, has scientific information taken precedence over the significance of human existence? In contrast, the spare embryos from clinical IVF programmes are the unrequired by-products of attempts to create new human life. By themselves, they cannot develop further, and so may be compared to naturally fertilized embryos that cannot develop further because of genetic abnormalities or hormonal deficiencies.

Fourth, requests to do research on human embryos should require especially strong justification because of the moral value accorded to each human embryo, and also to human embryos in general. In particular, research on human embryos should be considered only when no adequate substitute is available, and only to procure data likely to be of clinical importance. This emphasizes therapeutic research, at least as far as its value to embryos in general is concerned. Data of scientific interest alone should be obtained only using the embryos of experimental animals.

Fifth, the burden of demonstrating the acceptability of any proposed research should lie with those putting forward the proposal. Failure to provide convincing justification should be sufficient grounds for considering a proposal unacceptable. This is a built-in bias limiting research involving human embryos, and is a safeguard against premature or trivial proposals.

How, we may ask, can principles such as these be applied within society? It is not our intention to attempt to do this in any detail in this book, but we would argue that guidelines established and monitored by an official national bioethics committee (Jones and Telfer, 1990) are more appropriate than restrictive legislation (as in the state of Victoria in Australia). The difficulty with legislation in any rapidly-moving scientific area, especially when it touches on contentious scientific definitions, is that it just as rapidly becomes outdated or even anachronistic. Guidelines, by contrast, are open to community debate and can be modified as necessary. The one essential is that the guidelines must be enforceable.

Abortion

Of all ethical issues affecting life before birth, none are more daunting than those raised by abortion. The issues involved have become so polarized that the prospects of finding a consensus can appear forlorn. In some quarters, labels dominate every aspect of the debate with 'pro-life' and 'pro-choice' positions encapsulating all possible options within the two opposing perspectives. In other words, the vast complexity of moral discourse is whittled down to a simple decision — an absolute stance in favour of the unborn, or an absolute stance in favour of the mother's right to self-determination. Consequently, any mediating position is automatically placed in one or other of these categories.

In attempting to come to a workable ethical stance over abortion, we will suggest that account has to be taken of the wishes of the mother, the ethical demands made on us by the foetus, the relevance of the stage of foetal development, and the conflicting ethical assessment of abortion within society.

The first proposition we would defend is that abortion demands serious ethical assessment of the situation of both mother and foetus. To make decisions based on the interests of *only* mother *or* foetus is to deny the serious ethical weight that has to be placed on the personhood of the mother *and* on the potential for personhood of the foetus. This is necessary because, on the one hand, the mother is a person, whose bodily integrity should be respected and valued, but, on the other, since the (previable) foetus's continued existence is dependent upon its use of the mother's body, the mother's wishes regarding the uses to which her body should be put cannot be disregarded.

No matter how much protection we may wish to give the foetus, foetal protection cannot be absolute, since foetuses cannot be isolated from whatever conflicts are inherent in the human condition. Consequently, to expect complete protection for foetuses but less-than-complete protection for adults is to impose on foetuses an aura of idealism we do not impose on other members of the human community. Hence, there are occasions when the welfare of the foetus will come into conflict with the welfare of the mother, and ethical criteria have to be formulated for taking seriously the welfare of both. One of these criteria is, we consider, the extent of foetal maturity. We would argue that the degree of protection afforded the foetus should vary with the degree of foetal development increasing as development proceeds. From this it follows that a seven-month-old foetus should be provided with greater protection than a three-day-old embryo. This is because, in terms of a gradualist position, the former is closer to realising full personhood than is the latter (Poplawski and Gillett, 1991).

We suggest that foetal protection is to be abrogated where there is, or appears to be, unresolvable conflict. This will usually be between mother and foetus, although it may also involve the family unit, and it may be exacerbated by serious medical circumstances afflicting the foetus or the mother. The conflict ought to be of sufficient severity to jeopardize the health of mother and/or family. The level of potential harm will undoubtedly vary from one situation to another, depending on the social and religious culture in which the couple is living, and the degree of support available in the community in terms of the social and medical services available, and the help of family and friends.

We do not consider that the dilemma of abortion will be solved by restrictive legislation. This is due to the profound moral differences present within society. Many people are not persuaded that abortion is murder, and many consider that at certain stages during its development the foetus is a non-person. These are legitimate ethical perspectives that are incompatible with the belief that the embryo and foetus should be given absolute protection. Any attempt to enforce legislative restrictions on such people, when they have not been convinced by ethical arguments, is a dangerous way to proceed in a pluralist society.

Groups with firm ethical positions on the foetus, and therefore on abortion, have to appreciate the force of the ethical arguments of those with whom they disagree. This is particularly important for health workers, who have to deal as professionals with those having differing value systems. This conflict of values may arise between health professionals and patients, and highlights the obvious fact that doctors and nurses are also human beings with their own value systems. Some will regard abortion as equivalent to murder, and therefore will never be able to participate in abortion procedures with a clear conscience. For others, it will be no worse than removing an offending piece of tissue from a woman's body with her consent and they will feel quite easy about it.

Neither group should attempt to foist their own values on their patients, in an effort to safeguard their own moral autonomy. If their values conflict with those of their patients, they have an overriding obligation to ensure that the patient has access to alternative professional care.

Foetal neural transplantation

Foetal neural transplantation (brain grafting) burst upon the public scene in the late 1980s, and in so doing raised a host of ethical issues. In the flurry of activity surrounding this development, certain points were overlooked. The most immediate was that foetal *neural* transplantation is just one illustration of the transplantation of foetal tissues in general, all of which raise similar ethical considerations. Another point is that the use of *foetal* human tissues is just one illustration of the many uses society has made of human tissues and human material. The major reasons for considering foetal transplantation are for the alleviation of brain disease, such as Parkinson's disease, Alzheimer's disease, and Huntington's disease, and of Type 1 (juvenile) diabetes mellitus.

Since the focus of the foetal transplantation debate is the use of tissue from foetuses made available by induced abortion, particular attention needs to be paid to the dimensions of this debate. Four major positions can be recognized in relation to the significance of abortion for the foetal transplantation debate (Gillam, 1989).

1. Foetal tissue transplants are wrong, since experimental results to date are not good enough to warrant clinical application.

2. Foetal tissue transplants are wrong, because abortion is morally wrong and the wrongness of abortion cannot be isolated from any subsequent ethical decision concerning use of the foetal tissue.

3. Foetal tissue transplants are acceptable, because there is nothing morally wrong with abortion. Any safeguards that are required are to protect the woman having the abortion.

4. Foetal tissue transplants are acceptable, even if abortion is considered morally wrong. Such a separation is feasible because the two procedures are morally separate, as long as safeguards are in place to ensure that the abortion decision is kept separate from the transplant decision.

Position 1, that of *scientific pragmatism*, is familiar to everyone in clinical research (Jones, 1991). Premature use of new techniques or procedures, before they have been adequately worked out in laboratory research, is unethical. It is also unethical to carry out *ad hoc* clinical studies, in the absence of a clear protocol characterized by features such as standardization in patient selection and surgical technique, and rigorous follow-up among the centres performing the procedure in question. This position enshrines some important provisos, and yet it leaves the door open to future clinical developments. If these never eventuate, it will be for scientific, and not for ethical, reasons. It amounts, therefore, to a call for scientific and clinical judiciousness. In a few instances, it may result in a complete halt to all further developments.

Position 2 may be characterized as an *abortion-dependent* viewpoint, that stresses the moral abhorrence of abortion. This is such that it is regarded as tainting beyond acceptability any possible beneficial uses of the resulting foetal material. No separation of the two acts is seen to be possible, with the result that the deliberate killing of the foetus in the act of induced abortion renders anyone using material from such a foetus an accessory to premeditated killing. Generally associated with this position are fears that such uses of aborted material will lead to an increase in the rate of induced abortion in the community, and to women becoming pregnant in order to serve as a source of foetal material. Implicit within this position is an equality of status between foetus and mother, the result being that the foetus's interests are at least as important as those of the mother or patient. Any action that does not serve the foetus's interests is unethical, regardless of any good that may eventuate for others in the community.

Position 3, the *clinical benefit (abortion irrelevant)* stance, regards induced abortion as morally acceptable or, at least, of limited moral concern when placed alongside the potential benefits offered by such transplantation. Abortion may not, of necessity, be considered morally insignificant, but in weighing up the respective goods of a foetus unwanted by its mother (for whatever reasons) and of a patient capable of benefiting from foetal material, the balance in favour of the patient is unquestioned. Implicit within this viewpoint is a difference in the moral status of foetus and adult; that of the foetus is lower than that of both mother and patient. Restrictions are called for, but these reflect the mother's interests rather than those of the foetus.

Position 4 may be regarded as an *abortion-independent* position, and can be espoused even by those who view the foetus as a being deserving of profound respect based upon its potential for development into a fully-formed human person. Since the foetus is not to be treated as a mere object, a dead foetus is to be respected in the same manner as an adult human cadaver is respected. Consequently, following induced abortion foetal tissue can in principle be used in the same way as human organs are used for transplantation purposes following morally questionable or tragic circumstances. The thrust of this position depends entirely on the ability to view as morally acceptable a procedure (transplantation) that would not be possible apart from what many regard as a morally unacceptable procedure (induced abortion). Basic to this thrust is a complete separation in practice between the two procedures.

Having set out these four positions, the task is to decide how to assess their respective merits in a pluralist society. Of the four positions, the crucial one is probably the fourth, since it appears to reflect the stance of most within society. While it fails to encompass those at the two extremes of the moral spectrum, namely, those who view induced abortion as morally acceptable throughout most stages of foetal existence, and those who view abortion as morally reprehensible under all circumstances, the balancing of good and evil inherent within foetal transplantation pushes most people in the direction of the fourth position.

This position, however, has been criticized on grounds of moral complicity; that is, the transplantation fails to disentangle itself from the moral evil of the underlying abortion. According to this viewpoint, the use of aborted foetal tissue places the scientist in moral complicity with the person carrying out the abortion.

Moral complicity appears frequently in arguments over the use or otherwise of data and material emanating from the Nazi era, but appears to be ignored in discussions of other areas dependent upon the use of human material. These include discussions of the means employed to obtain a supply of human bodies for dissection in the eighteenth and nineteenth centuries (see Chapter 3), the source of human embryos and foetuses for the study of normal human development, and the source of organs for organ transplantation in adults.

The problem with the moral complicity argument is that it proves too strong. It is generally used selectively, when abortion or Nazi atrocities are involved. However, it is not limited to these. If human tissue is used from any source, there is almost inevitably complicity in some moral evil. This may be complicity in the road toll when organs are used from the victims of automobile accidents, in homicide when organs are used from murder victims, in suicide when organs are used from those who have committed suicide, or in poverty when the cadavers of the destitute are used for dissection. To suggest that the surgeon or anatomist is in a supportive alliance with intoxicated car drivers, murderers, those who commit suicide, or an inequitable social system bears little relationship to moral reality. There *is* a moral distance between the evil and the intended good, although this can readily be eroded. However, if the significance of this distance is rejected, most uses of human material become unethical and most medically-related disciplines automatically become tainted with moral evil.

We act routinely on the assumption that good can come from evil. As a general principle, we are prepared to benefit from tragedies, and this is regarded as an ethically valid stance as long as we are in no way responsible for the tragedies, and if we would have prevented them had we been in a position to do so. For instance, many studies of malnourished children have thrown a great deal of light on the effects of malnutrition on the developing brain, while studies of the after-effects of the atom bomb explosions at Hiroshima and Nagasaki have proved of enormous value in understanding the long-term effects of radiation on human populations. As societies, we are prepared to benefit from tragedies, with the one proviso that the killing and maiming are not undertaken in order to yield scientific data.

The study and use of human material are implicit within medicine. There is no way of avoiding this, and there is no way of avoiding research on human persons. The ethical question, therefore, is not whether this should be done, but how it should be done. The use of human material is not always justified, but it is sometimes justified. The framework to be erected is that of balancing the needs and aspirations of *this* human being upon whom research is being conducted or who is being used for therapeutic purposes, against the needs and aspirations of *that* human being who is expected to benefit from the research or therapy.

Certain predominant principles appear to be emerging. These are clearly expressed by the 1989 report of the Polkinghorne Committee (Review of Guidance on the Research Use of Fetuses and Fetal Material, 1989) in Britain on the use of foetuses and foetal material. It stated: 'Central to our understanding is the acceptance of a special status for the living human fetus at every stage of its development into a fully-formed human being. The fetus is not to be treated instrumentally as a mere object available for investigation or use. That respect carries over in a modified fashion to the dead fetus, in a way analogous to the respect we afford a human cadaver on the basis of its having been the body of a human person.'

After considering objections to foetal transplantation on the basis of the morally objectionable nature of induced abortion, the Committee continues: 'The situation . . . is one in which a number of possible conflicting moral factors are involved. We do not believe that in circumstances of such moral complexity it is right to regard the termination of pregnancy as inevitably so heinous that any subsequent use of the fetal tissue thereby made available is morally disqualified.'

Principles such as these have been seen as leading to certain guidelines in practice. The major ones (Jones, 1989) are that:

1. The foetus must be dead; with the tissue being taken from a foetal cadaver.
2. The abortion is not to be influenced in any way by the prospect of foetal grafting, its manner and timing being unaffected by such procedures.
3. The abortion and the grafting are to be kept completely separate.

Additional guidelines include:

1. There is a genuine possibility of significant benefit to a specific patient or patients suffering from a specific (neurological) disease.
2. The good expected from the therapy or research is greater than any harm that might be attached to the use of aborted foetuses.
3. This form of therapy is used as a last resort, all conventional forms of therapy having been found inadequate.
4. There is fully informed consent of the pregnant woman to any procedures that might affect her, and appropriate consent (proxy consent according to some writers) for the use of foetal material.
5. The recipient is in a position to provide fully informed consent.
6. There is anonymity between donor and recipient, excluding the possibility of any relationship between them.
7. The research design should be sound so that the study contributes in a substantial way to ongoing understanding of the grafting procedure of the diseases involved.

Together, these guidelines take account of all relevant ethical principles, providing protection for all the parties involved in the transplantation procedure. Differences of opinion will still occur but, as we have seen, these revolve around the most basic (some would say irreconcilable) ethical questions. The most that guidelines like these can do is allow others to act in ethically appropriate ways.

Chapter 5

Neonatal and childhood issues

A child is born with a severe form of cri-du-chat syndrome. Against medical advice, the parents request that the heart defect be corrected. This is done and some months later the child is admitted to a paediatric chronic care institution where she is unresponsive apart form occasional mewing cries.

Our impulse in medicine is to furnish help and comfort to the human beings who come to us, and to do so by using whatever technology is appropriate. The ill child makes an asymmetrical appeal for love and care, and cannot repay that except by responding to the attitudes that we show. Our care for the human infant is an expression of our membership of a human community in which the dependant members call for our protection. If we were to suppress this deep commitment to members of our own species, we would undermine one of the natural well-springs of moral understanding, therefore we acknowledge a creative responsibility for the development of the 'little person' concerned.

However, there are some groups of children about whose potential we must think more carefully before we allow our moral concern to result in heroic medicine. First, there are children who do not have any conscious appreciation of life and will never develop it. They have the physical appearance of human beings, but lack the essential functional qualities of being human which include the capacity for conscious life. These children do not function at a level that is basic to participation with others as a being to whom things matter, and they never will function at that level. If an individual can show neither any awareness of, nor response to, the care and love of other human beings, then we would seem to be on fairly safe ground in concluding the individual is not equipped to appreciate things as mattering to it. Where there is neither the capacity nor the potential for personal life, our normal medical concern to treat for recovery can be appropriately suppressed. Such children will include those with microcephaly, anencephaly, hydrancncephaly, and certain other major CNS deformities. Whenever we can say that the children concerned have been born without the potential to enter into human relations, we could say that we are released from any obligation to keep them alive.

What of children who do have some capacity for participation in human relationships, but have such severe handicaps that intervention seems to gain little more than prolonged suffering? Often, the decision is made to offer no treatment, apart from basic comfort and custodial care, because anything more would be cruel and fruitless if inflicted on the being concerned. This is the issue confronting those involved in the decision-making about the child with cri-du-chat syndrome. What was gained for anyone in the intervention to correct a heart defect, except (perhaps) some reassurance to the parents that they had done all that they could for their child? When intervention also becomes the prolongation of suffering, such a reason should not be the determinative one. Instead, concern for the child must prevail.

> Alice was born with oxalosis. By the age of two she had developed stones in the kidneys and increasingly severe renal failure. For some weeks she drifted in and out of uraemic coma with her parameters being carefully monitored and adjusted by zealous junior paediatric staff. Each day she needed blood tests to check for electrolytes and acid base regulation. Each few days she needed her IV lines renewed and these were increasingly difficult to site. She was usually in pain and her small body was pale and weak. It was eventually decided, in consultation with her parents, to let her drift into uraemic coma and die.

If such decisions are morally justified, should there be a more forthright determination on the part of paediatricians and parents to eliminate handicap by much more rigorously selective treatment policies, or indeed by painlessly killing those who are defective in any serious sense?

> A slightly older couple look forward to their first child, only to be devastated when the child has Down's syndrome. They refuse to authorize surgery for duodenal atresia, but they are overridden by the courts and the surgery is performed. Years later they are still having difficulties accepting that their child will not achieve the educational and other goals that they had hoped for, but they love him very much.

A number of philosophers have suggested that it is only a sentimental 'speciesism' which brings about such restrictive judgements on parental wishes. For example, Peter Singer, in an essay on sanctity versus quality of life (Singer, 1983), argues that it is merely the fact that such defective infants are members of the species *homo sapiens* that makes the imposition of treatment different from what defective dogs or pigs would receive. If we were concerned more rationally with the balance of happiness over suffering, we would not prolong defective human lives needlessly. Singer's challenge forces us to examine more carefully the principled basis for the special concern for the lives of young and helpless human beings who suffer from handicaps.

How can we defend the idea that the ethical importance of a human being is greater than that of other animals? We stand accused that this judgement is just an irrational prejudice in favour of our own species. To meet the challenge, we usually invoke facts about the wishes and desires of the individuals concerned, their conscious appreciation of life, and/or their preferences about what should happen to them. But, on any set of criteria of this type, it is plain to see that neonates, possibly infants, and arguably certain mentally defective children, turn out to be less well-qualified candidates for ethical consideration than animals such as chimpanzees, gorillas, perhaps dolphins, and even pigs!

It is, however, unacceptable to be told not to grieve about the death of an infant or neonate, because it does not really matter any more than the death of a valued family pet. Our concern for other humans goes deeper than mere regard for species membership — it is a fundamental part of our nature as ethical beings. Certain reactions, sensitivities, and responses are the basis of moral judgements. Moral reasoning concerns evaluative concepts that are learned through human relationships and which involve the understanding of suffering. A person grasps the types of wishes and needs that others have, because his own desires and needs are enunciated in concepts that are learned through his interactions with others. Thus, he has a tendency to empathy toward others just because they are human; this natural empathy underlies many of his moral sensitivities. Without empathy of this very natural type, and the feelings of compassion to which it leads, a person would not 'catch on' to the reasons why moral considerations are important. Therefore, although we can argue about what is the right thing to do, we also depend on a feeling that certain things are right and that a tendency to do right things and not to do wrong things should constrain our choices.

Another natural response is to take care of the young of one's species. This, too, is part of that foundation in human nature on which moral understanding is built. To harm a child or to exercise wanton cruelty toward another human being betrays a basic ingredient in our ability to make any moral judgements at all. If one does not feel the force of the moral imperatives concerning children, then one is impaired in one's moral thinking. That is why the death of a child, no matter how young, is a shocking tragedy. We find our noblest and most creatively altruistic tendencies enlisted in our response to children. In a way, all that is best in oneself finds a focus in the appeal of a child. To the shock of death is added the loss of that possibility of sharing and of being a better person, of watching a life unfold and respond to what one has to give.

Yet are there not circumstances in which we should carry the responsibility of a child's death as a necessary and humane action? Ironically, the sanctity with which we endow all human life often works to the detriment of those unfortunate humans whose lives hold no prospect except suffering. Singer is right to the extent that, while a dog or pig, dying slowly and painfully, will be mercifully released from its misery, a human being in similar circumstances may well have to endure its hopeless condition until the end.

> A nine-month-old child develops vomiting and rapidly becomes unconscious after a minor flu-like illness. The diagnosis is Reye syndrome. She continues to worsen to the point where cerebral circulation is compromised. She has clinical brain death except for occasional extensor spasms and swallowing movements. Respirator and nasogastric feeding support continue for months until the decision is made to turn off the ventilator.

What was the right action to take in this and similar situations? A full consideration of this issue must await our discussion of euthanasia (see Chapter 8). A preliminary answer may be attempted in terms of the fundamental orientation of medicine toward the saving or salvaging of human lives, an orientation which can lead to over-meddlesome medicine, but whose elimination could well be a greater threat to human well-being. Doctors and nurses persevere in what can be a very demanding professional task because of a powerful presumption in favour of preserving or restoring life. Faced with a human being whose form has been distorted or defaced, the medical reaction is to expend extraordinary effort on behalf of that individual. The successes of medicine throughout history have been inspired by this impulse. Conversely, to kill or deliberately neglect an individual who is afflicted is to obey a fundamentally different impulse. A medical profession which over-treats out of misplaced therapeutic zeal is certainly to be deplored, but a less ethically admirable approach to paediatric medicine would be one which coldly seeks to eliminate handicap. Between these two extremes responsible choices must be made, choices focused on the best interests of the individual child as far as we can predict and assess them.

Parental decisions regarding treatment options

In most jurisdictions there is a fuzzy boundary between the age at which a child can give consent to her own treatment and the age at which parental consent must be sought. Most ethicists advise that the child be included as far as possible in the decision-making process but for children up to at least sixteen years old, the parents should give consent to medical treatment.

The basis for the parental right to choose treatment for children rests in the intuition that parents are protectors of the child and responsible for the child's care. This is regarded as the 'natural role' of parents and is recognized universally in legal codes. It is assumed that the parent is training and nurturing the child to bring that child to the point where she can make her own decisions. We act on the presumption that the parents will make decisions in the best interests of the child and, on this basis, empower them to do so. However, in certain situations, this presumption cannot be sustained.

> Anna is a five-year-old girl with a heart defect. She requires surgery in which blood will be recirculated and a transfusion may be given to her. Her parents object on religious grounds to her receiving any blood. The surgeon and physicians involved believe that she will die without surgery and that surgery cannot be performed without blood being given. The petition is made to the Court and the child is made a ward of the court for the duration of her treatment because the court believes that the parents are not acting in the best interests of the child.

This decision shows what we believe to be paramount in dilemmas involving children. We believe that the child's interests should come first. In Anna's case that meant overturning parental authority because it was felt their judgement was distorted by their religious belief so that they could not rightly discern the best interests of the child.

Special problems arise with high-risk neonates whose quality of life may well be compromised and for whom many would incline towards a 'compassionate' refusal to keep the child alive. The ethical problems here are many. The overwhelming tendency of the law is not to get involved but to rely on co-operative decisions by parents and clinicians. Here we must consider: (a) the moral limits on parental choice; (b) the need to lighten the load of responsibility and guilt on parents for a life and death choice; and (c) the need to be sensitive to the limits of one's medical responsibility and not play God in the lives of others, not only in medical decisions, but also in the social and long-term commitments of those decisions. Parents must not be forced to suffer a burden of responsibility, and perhaps guilt, for a decision that we should be prepared to share. They must be helped to do what is right in such a way as they do not feel that they have the role of arbiters of life and death for the child they have produced.

Child abuse and child protection

Sometimes the presumption of parental care is mistaken.

> Dion is eighteen months old. He is admitted with fits, vomiting, and irritability. On examining him, the doctors find that he has haemorrhages in his retina and bruises on his limbs, with a superficially infected burn on his foot. A CT scan reveals a chronic left-sided subdural haematoma and a skeletal survey shows a healing fracture of the left humerus and broken ribs on the right side. The doctors interview the mother and her live-in partner. Social Welfare are informed and the child protection team comes to see the child who is made a ward of court. Burrholes are performed to remove the subdural haematoma.

The likely course of events in this case is that the child will be removed from the custody of the mother until the child protection team can take steps to remove the danger to Dion, and assure themselves that Dion will not suffer by being returned to his mother's care. She may have a part in this decision but she will not be authorized to make decisions for the child, as she has failed in the role of guardian. There may, of course, be reasons for her actions or for her allowing someone to injure the child, but these are not material to decisions about the welfare of the child in the short term. The short-term priority is to protect the child from harm and to act in the child's best interests. Long-term interests can be regarded as soon as it is clear that the child is safe and unlikely to be more damaged than he already has been by the physical abuse he has received.

All of these decisions are difficult and require careful judgement. The doctor must take special precautions in dealing with child abuse cases. A colleague ought always to be called upon (where this is possible) to validate findings and confirm the decision. Those with the responsibility for overall care must give, in particular, very careful consideration to the diagnosis and its evidential base. Social Welfare ought to be involved as soon as the diagnosis is clear. In this situation, information gained by the doctor is not under the normal confidentiality constraints. It can and should be shared with those who are entrusted with the child's protection. Prior to their involvement, it should be used to provide sufficient reason for the need for their involvement to be established.

The health care professional should be aware of the tangled loyalties and dynamics of these situations. A doctor, nurse, or social worker may well feel committed to and sorry for a young, perhaps disadvantaged, mother of a child like Dion. This mother may well be as needy as her child, and the health care professional may look upon her as a client requiring special support. This should not be allowed to cloud the issue of the best interests of the child. Once the child is safe from harm, the situation can be addressed more calmly and deliberately than is possible in the 'messy' period when suspicions abound and nothing has been done to bring the problem to the attention of those whose expertise is needed. Often, by taking things out of the hands of the non-coping parent(s), the doctor can relieve the guilt and tension in the fraught and complex situation. In any event we must recognize, in cases of child abuse, that our loyalties clearly lie with more than one person, and that the person most at risk is also the person least likely to be able to safeguard his own interests. Dion runs significant risks of death or permanent disability, and because it is the persons who nature and society expect to protect him that are themselves the source of his danger, he needs our full protection.

The 'best interests of the child' criterion

The problems surrounding child abuse highlight the fact that children are not possessions of their parents but human individuals, persons in the process of becoming persons in their own right. Thus we have to weigh the wishes of parents against what is best for the child wherever there is reason to believe that they are not in full agreement. There are not many situations where this is the case. Often parents will see more clearly than doctors that a child has had enough and that some 'heroic' treatment should be discontinued. (In this they are often supported by nurses who are closest to the child in day-by-day clinical care.) However, there are situations where the parents will be so upset by what has happened or is happening to their child that they will not make a good decision.

> Barbara is a twelve-year-old girl who is brought into hospital having collapsed at home. She is found to have had a haemorrhage in her right occipital lobe. By the time she is stabilized it is clear that she is beginning to develop a right temporal pressure cone with dilatation of the right pupil and a steady deterioration in her conscious level as measured by the Glasgow Coma Score. An angiogram is performed which shows an AV malformation based in the right lateral ventricle of the brain. The need for an operation to save her life, the fact that she has partially lost her sight, and the risk of some residual damage to the brain are all explained rather hurriedly to the parents in seeking their consent for urgent operation.

Barbara is a very attractive girl and, when they are faced by these rather dire prospects (although it is mentioned that her long-term prospects are good) and the need for her to have her head shaved for a brain operation, both parents, the mother most vehemently, say that they cannot consent to surgery and that she should be allowed to die in peace. Words like 'brain damage', 'vegetable', 'like a horror camp victim', and so on, punctuate their discussion. The doctors and nurses try to reason with them but to no avail. Eventually, having informed their Chief Medical Officer, they go ahead with the operation. The medical officer informs the local child protection team and the child is in the process of being made a ward of court when an uncle, brother of Barbara's mother, contacts the medical team to say that the parents will sign consent for surgery.

In this situation the health care team were forced to an extreme measure to save the life of a girl who would almost certainly fare very well despite her urgent neurosurgical problem. It is likely that she will have a partial visual defect, but otherwise her vision will be intact and she will function normally. It would certainly be wrong to concur with a decision in which emotional disturbance would cost this girl her life.

Libby is thirteen. Her parents are separated because of problems between them and related problems involving sexual abuse of Libby and her nine-year-old sister. Libby has a relapsing leukaemia which has escaped three cycles of chemotherapy and produced a malignant meningitis also unresponsive to intrathecal care. Libby and her mother had decided that comfort measures were all she could cope with, and the paediatric oncologist agreed. The father contacted the superintendent and said that if anything less than full active treatment measures were used he would see that the Health Board and the doctors involved were sued for manslaughter. He demanded to see his daughter and, after an emotional scene, Libby tearfully decided she had to keep fighting.

Here, we need to be especially aware of the strain put on Libby by the wider dynamics of her situation. It would seem that the health care professionals involved, particularly female professionals, need to get very close to Libby so as to enable her to make authentic and undistorted decisions about her own future. It would be unlikely, in this situation, that the father's legal threats would get very far but, on all sides, the decisions would be more secure if discussions were clearly documented, at least in outline, and clear medical and ethical reasons given for the choices made.

Resource allocation and at-risk children

The special regard in which we hold children can lead to unwise resource allocation decisions. It is often possible to obtain large amounts of money by using graphic portrayals of the plight of sick children. This can mean that health care resources are not, in the larger picture, used wisely. To avoid this we need to bear in mind several crucial points affecting resource allocation to paediatrics.

1. Money spent is not always to meet a one-off cost as often the intervention prevents or mitigates complications that would later be very costly in health care terms.

> The neonatal unit was threatened with a cut to funding so that they could not treat as many children. They had two choices — they could accept an overall budgetary constraint or else accept a handed-down policy of non-treatment for all children under 750 grams. They pointed out that the latter policy would mean that over three years, approximately one child who might survive with some disability, would instead die. This saving was thought to be minuscule compared with the overall throughput. It was also pointed out that most of the under 750 gram children who actually survived did so with a good quality of life and the policy would condemn these children to die. It was finally pointed out that there were children of birthweight greater than 750 grams who ought not to be treated, and yet the policy would implicitly mandate that such children should receive treatment regardless. The alternative was to ensure the informed joint decisions made by parents and the neonatal team, and encourage cessation of treatment where the prognosis was hopeless in children of any birthweights.

This example suggests that informed conjoint decisions should remain the cornerstone of health care policy for neonates: parents must be given realistic prognoses, and the option of care, but not heroic intervention, should be endorsed for those children who fall into the two categories outlined above (those who will never achieve conscious life and those who will experience little except suffering). This is a far more sensitive response to shortages of funds than heavy-handed lines drawn across the continuum of birthweights or other parameters.

2. Spectacular reports from centres in other parts of the world can often prompt a dramatic appeal for some new and unproven therapy for a child with a tragic condition. This kind of drama often works to the detriment of other sick children in terms of reduced funding across the board, and therefore reduced opportunity costs for other areas of paediatric care.

The correct ethical response to such an appeal is a careful and measured consideration of the costs and benefits of the proposed high profile therapy, and a diligent consideration of local and often cheaper but equally effective alternatives. If this were done by honest, unbiased medical opinion which was open-minded enough to give alternatives a fair hearing, then much misleading optimism and disappointment would be avoided. The almost hysterical playing on our natural sympathy for children, that sometimes occurs, can only be destructive in the long term and costly for the community concerned. What is more, it threatens the credibility of real medical advances for suffering children. Health care professionals in particular ought to be aware of this danger, and alert to the abuses to which it gives rise.

Children as research participants

Finally, we come to a topic which will be more fully dealt with in the next chapter: the use of human beings as participants in research projects. The general issues associated with research will be discussed later but, in the case of children, a fundamental dilemma arises: unless the research project can be shown to be of direct benefit to the child (and this would be a rare circumstance), has anyone the right to enlist a child in the project? In all other situations of consent on behalf of children, the presumption is that the guiding principle is the best interests of the child. How can a parent — or any other person — volunteer a child for procedures which are not for the child's benefit, and which may carry an element of risk?

One way of dealing with this difficulty is to insist that, whatever the legal age for consent, a child should always be consulted about research participation, and no action should be taken to which the child does not give clear assent. This is only a partial solution, however. In the first place, a significant proportion of paediatric research is carried out on neonates, or on children well below the age of understanding. Moreover, even when a child is old enough to be given an explanation, the scope of comprehension may be quite limited, and the influence of parents or other significant adults on the decision-making process will be considerable. One cannot make young children into the equivalent of adult volunteers.

This leaves two options: to ban all non-therapeutic research on infants and young children; or to find some other form of moral justification. If a ban is to be avoided, then we must develop a broader view of 'benefit' than that which views only direct benefit to that individual child to be a legitimizing factor. We all, both adults and children, have an interest in the progress of medicine through the application of well-designed and effective research. Children, in particular, have an interest in the progress of paediatric medicine, and would be harmed by a ban which prevented whole areas of that field from being adequately researched. Thus, although a specific project might be of no conceivable benefit to the individual child participating as a research subject, the prevention of all such forms of research could well present a hazard. For example, the child acting as a control subject in a study of asthmatic children may never need therapy for this form of respiratory disorder, but could well benefit from an improved understanding of therapeutic measures in paediatric respiratory medicine generally.

Taking this broader view, we may countenance the involvement of children in research, provided some stringent conditions are observed. Firstly, it can never be justifiable to volunteer another to undergo any significant risk for what can be only a very indirect benefit. Thus, all paediatric research (of no direct benefit to the research subjects) must carry minimal or negligible risk. In assessing such risks, the dangers of creating anxiety or embarrassment in young children must also be avoided.

Secondly, parental consent to participation of a child does not of itself legitimize a research project. There is a special responsibility on the researcher, and on those committees vetting the research, to ensure that the project is well designed, safe, and worth doing. Parents may not be in a position to assess this fully and objectively, and may be predisposed to co-operation out of a sense of indebtedness to the medical institutions caring for their child.

Thirdly, every effort should be made to make the child into a research *participant* rather than merely a passive recipient of procedures which he cannot understand. Even if valid consent cannot be obtained, the active involvement of the child should be sought where possible, and research should never be allowed to proceed when the child is clearly distressed by the procedures.

Finally, no research which could equally well be done on adults should ever be done on children. Children should never be used merely because they are accessible (e.g. as patients in an institution) and reasonably compliant. Research with children as participants should be research especially necessary for the welfare of children. In this way, we begin to teach children the mutual obligations within which we live, and help them to recognize that special form of identification with the needs of others which leads to altruism. The child who learns to care for the sufferings of other children is much more than a mere research subject. The experience becomes a source of learning about the purpose of research and the meaning of the medical enterprise as a whole.

Thus, as we have been stressing throughout this chapter, there is much to be learned from paediatric medicine about the basic moral values which underlie medicine as a whole. When we learn to respect the vulnerability of children, and to enhance the development of their capacities as autonomous moral agents, we see the humanistic roots of medicine from which the whole endeavour of health care gains its stability and strength.

Chapter 6

Medical research

At the conclusion of World War Two the full horrors of life in institutions for the intellectually handicapped and in the concentration camps of the Third Reich were revealed to public view. Among other atrocities, the Nuremberg Trials revealed that doctors had, in the name of science, performed mutilating and totally experimental gynaecological operations on female inmates, and had tested the limits of human survival at low temperatures by immersing prisoners in baths of icy water. The philosophy underlying these actions was that certain classes of human being were totally expendable, of no individual worth, but merely the means to some alleged 'common good'. Since these revelations four decades ago, the topic of scientific experimentation using human subjects has been seen as one in which the ethical issues are clear and unambiguous. Whatever the benefits which might be gained from the use of human beings as experimental subjects, there cannot be any justification for treating people as mere means to an end. The rights of the individual remain paramount, and no scientific advance can outweigh the harm done by unethical research. Yet, even after all these years, there are still areas where some uncertainty remains (though not at the barbarous level of the Nazi experiments), in terms of the balance to be achieved between worthy social goals and individual rights.

The basic principles guiding research with human subjects were firmly enunciated in the Nuremberg Code, drawn up at the conclusion of the War Crime Trials. The code stressed the necessity of gaining fully informed consent from subjects, the obligation on the researcher to ensure that there were no undue risks, and that any minimal risks were clearly outweighed by the benefits to be gained. Although this code was promulgated in 1947, its application to biomedical research was not always perceived. There was no repetition of the Nazi atrocities; however some medical research was carried out in the post-war era which did entail risks to subjects, of which they were not informed. In the early 1960s awareness of this lack of ethical supervision in medical research was growing, particularly as a result of the writings of

M.H. Pappworth (*Human Guinea Pigs*) and H.K. Beecher (*Research and the Individual*). The World Medical Association prepared a draft code of ethics relating to human experimentation in 1962, which, after wide circulation and comment, was adopted by the WMA Assembly meeting in Helsinki in 1965. The Helsinki Declaration, which has subsequently gone through several revisions (the latest one being in 1989), forms the basis for the ethical monitoring and control of medical research worldwide. The examples of unethical research which follow will demonstrate why a clear enunciation of principles and guidelines was needed.

> In 1957, an experimental programme was introduced in the Willowbrook Hospital, an institution for intellectually handicapped children in New York State. Numerous infections were rife in the hospital, including viral hepatitis. The researchers set up a special unit in which selected children were deliberately infected with the virus in order to study the course of the disease. The researchers argued that, since the children would probably be infected anyway, they were better off in the special unit than in the general wards of the hospital.

But this calculation of harm versus benefit is sustainable only if no attempt were made to improve the hygiene and level of infection in the hospital as a whole. Moreover, parents giving consent to the admission of their children to the unit were in effect coerced into their decision by being warned that the alternative was likely infection without sustained medical attention. Thus, a vulnerable group was induced to participate in a research programme which under normal circumstances would never attract any volunteers.

In the next example, the intention to benefit the subjects is much clearer, but there was no proper assessment of the risks to subjects, and a complete failure to gain informed consent to participation.

> In 1966, a research proposal was instituted in National Women's Hospital, Auckland, which was designed to demonstrate that carcinoma *in situ*, a symptomless lesion in the cervix, was not (as had been hitherto thought) a precursor to invasive carcinoma. The proposal entailed taking no action to excise the abnormal area, but rather following up the women at regular intervals to determine whether there were any signs of progression. As the subsequent judicial enquiry (the Cartwright Enquiry) showed, this was a risky, poorly designed experiment which led to unnecessary disease (in some cases fatal) in a number of subjects. Moreover, none of the women involved were ever made aware that they were participating in an unusual and experimental treatment; the need for frequent return visits for checking was both an inconvenience for them, and — in those cases in which invasive cancer developed — a false reassurance.

These two examples illustrate how important it is for medical researchers to be aware of the fundamental ethical principles governing research with human beings, and to establish proper procedures for assessing and monitoring the ethical aspects of research projects. We shall look at the application of the basic principles under the following headings: scientific validity; risk versus benefit; informed consent; and procedures for ensuring the ethical conduct of research.

Scientific validity

A research proposal cannot be ethical if it lacks scientific validity. Poorly designed research entails putting subjects at risk or, at the least, to some inconvenience, for no clear benefit. This means that every proposal to undertake research must be subjected to scientific assessment, to determine whether there is a clear hypothesis to be tested and to make sure that the research design will yield the result sought after. When research is supported by major funding bodies such as the Health Research Council of New Zealand, this assessment will be carried out as a matter of course before any grant is awarded. When research is commercially funded (e.g. by pharmaceutical companies) an independent assessment of the research proposal must be made to determine whether any useful and *new* information will be gained, or whether what is claimed to be 'research' is in fact a marketing exercise (e.g. designed to draw the attention of general practitioners to a particular brand of drug). If a research project is carried out by an individual without reference to any external funding body, then scientific assessment will be an integral part of the decision about whether there are ethical objections to its implementation. Poorly designed research is at best a waste of research participants' time, at worst a subjecting of people to unnecessary risk. We may say, without doubt, that bad science is also bad ethics.

Even if a research project is scientifically valid, it may not be justifiable. In some instances, the research may merely be going over old ground which has already been covered by previous research. In other instances, the information to be gained may be of little obvious use or benefit to anyone. Thus the question should be asked of every proposed research, would anything be lost if this project did *not* proceed? This question need not be answered in a too narrowly pragmatic sense. Much research is contributing to fundamental scientific understanding of processes without any practical advantage being immediately evident. It is, however, on such well researched foundations that future practical applications of science will be based. But whenever human subjects are involved, it is essential to avoid what can be seen as trivial or permanently insignificant and pointless research. Once again, a proper scientific assessment can establish the relationship of the proposed research to other work in the field and to current promising lines of development.

Risks and benefits

Once the general scientific viability of the project has been established, the relative balance of risks and benefits must be assessed. The Declaration of Helsinki has drawn a basic distinction between therapeutic and non-therapeutic research. The former may be of direct or indirect benefit to the subjects since it consists in improving knowledge either about the diseased condition of the subjects or about possible improvements in therapy for their condition. For example, a surgeon may wish to try out a new operative technique, or a physician may wish to test a new drug, using as research subjects a group of patients under her care.

In therapeutic research, the main guideline to be followed is that, without the research, there could be no certainty about which of the interventions being tested will be of greater benefit to the patient. In these circumstances, it is justifiable to randomize patients to one treatment or another, since, until the research is complete, one cannot tell whether the patients being given the new treatment, or the patients not being given it, will benefit more. Of course, if there is reasonable evidence that harm could be caused to one group, then the research should never begin. The basic principle in medical care is that each patient should be given the best treatment available for that particular condition, and that harm should never be knowingly caused (*primum non nocere*). One cannot justify withholding a treatment of known benefit to patients merely in the interests of research.

It is obvious that in some therapeutic trials there will be an element of risk for subjects. For example, in order to test a new drug for hypertension, there would have to be a weaning-off period in which a placebo is administered, prior to the administration of the drug to the experimental group. To ensure validity, this would have to be undertaken 'blinded' to both researchers and research subjects. Risks of this kind, created by the design of the trial itself, can be dealt with only by very thorough procedures for monitoring the medical condition of subjects in order to give immediate warning of when it will be necessary to break the code in order to give appropriate treatment to the person affected. A research design is acceptable only when the safety of subjects throughout the trial period is the paramount concern.

In non-therapeutic research, when there is no anticipated advantage to the subjects (apart perhaps from the satisfaction of assisting in the advance of medical knowledge), the protection of the rights of subjects must again be of paramount importance. For example, researchers might wish to improve their understanding of the mechanisms of conception by obtaining samples of uterine tissue from post-menopausal women. The procedure involved (biopsy) has a very low risk, but could cause some discomfort and could be embarrassing for some women. Yet participation in such a project could only be from purely altruistic motives, since reproductive capacity is no longer relevant to that group. We must, therefore, be sure that subjects are fully informed of the nature of the research, especially of the precise nature of the sampling procedures, so that they are not in any way coerced into taking part.

When subjects are enlisted as controls in a therapeutic trial, that aspect of the trial is non-therapeutic research. For example, research into children with behavioural problems might include as controls a group of children who were known not to have such problems. Since there is no benefit to such subjects, risks which might otherwise be thought to be quite minor (e.g. inconvenience or the causing of embarrassment or transient anxiety) assume greater importance. Some writers believe that subjects who are incapable of giving informed consent (e.g. very young children) should never be enlisted in non-therapeutic research, because proxy decisions are not justifiable for procedures of no clear benefit to such subjects (see the fuller discussion of this issue in Chapter 5). But this rigorous standard would in effect bring to a halt all research in paediatrics, and much research in psychiatry and geriatrics. The alternative to this absolutist view is to insist that the risk must be so minimal as to be negligible in all circumstances where the consent of the subject cannot be obtained. In assessing risk, account must be taken not only of possible physical injury but of levels of discomfort, inconvenience, anxiety, or invasion of privacy. The more intrusive the research, the less justification can be offered for enlisting individuals who cannot assess the risks for themselves.

Information and consent

In all types of research, whether therapeutic or non-therapeutic, the provision of comprehensive and accurate information to subjects, or their proxy decision-makers, is crucial. Without such information, the consent granted will not be valid. Giving informed consent is not to be confused with the signing of a consent form. This should merely be the formal acknowledgment of a process whereby the person giving consent has come to a full understanding of what is entailed, has been made aware that there is complete freedom either to grant or withhold consent, and that the consent may be withdrawn at any stage in the research. To achieve this fully valid form of consent, great attention must be paid to the quality of the communication about the project. All explanations must be in non-technical and readily understood language, and (except in the most trivial circumstances) be provided in a written as well as a spoken form. The information should include a clear description of any risks and an assurance that refusal to participate will in no way alter the medical care the subject is receiving.

In addition to adequate information, valid consent requires that subjects are not coerced or induced into participation. Subjects in a special relationship to the researcher (e.g. as patients or students) can be protected from coercion by the use of independent third parties (e.g. nurses not connected with the ward or department) to seek consent. Payments to subjects (which are substantial enough to constitute an inducement) invalidate consent. In practice, it may be hard to distinguish between payments which are described as a refund of expenses and recompense for the inconvenience, and what is in effect a bribe to take part. A total ban on payments, on the other hand, may prevent much useful research taking place. Certainly, where there is any risk to subjects or where the subjects themselves are vulnerable because of their impoverished condition, the ethical justification of paying research subjects is very dubious. The volunteer relationship in medical research seems much more securely based ethically, since it gives the research subject a sense of partnership in the project. A serious danger in all research is that the subject is treated merely as a means to an end, rather than as a freely participating moral agent.

It is because of this emphasis on respect for the person of the research subject, that only in exceptional circumstances is it justifiable to omit to gain consent. An absence of risk to the subject is not a justification in itself.

> Two researchers in a medical school want to do a study on the placentas of primigravida women. They submit a proposal to an ethical committee which outlines what they are intending to do but contains no consent form, since (they claim) consent is unnecessary in view of the fact that the placentas would be incinerated anyway. What harm then would there be in a few tests on them first?

Consent is necessary in such a case because although the tissue is of no further use to the individual, it is that person's right to determine how it shall be used. Failure to give full information and to gain consent betrays a lack of respect for the women concerned; they are being treated as sources of useful research material, rather than as potential partners in a project whose value they could appreciate. Moreover, there is a possibility of harm in the case of those women who, for cultural or religious reasons, would regard such a use of the products of birth as disrespectful or distasteful. The same strictures must apply to the use of any tissue removed at operation.

We can see, then, that consent is important, not only because it signifies that the participants in research have been given the opportunity to make their own assessment of the risks and benefits, but because the consent process recognizes that the research subject is a person in her own right, with a set of personal values which must be respected. Research without consent constitutes an invasion of the personal integrity of the research subjects, even if no physical harm is caused to them.

The situations in which the omission of consent (or proxy consent) is permissible are those in which totally non-invasive procedures are proposed, and the obtaining of consent would be impractical or possibly even alarming to the subjects. These conditions sometimes arise in epidemiological research. For example, the following arguments have been put forward for responsible accessing of medical records under certain circumstances.

> Research into the incidence of cancer in certain groups (e.g. those in specific occupations) may entail following up hospital records over a number of years to identify risk factors. It would not be possible to contact all the subjects to obtain consent for access to their records, because of changes of address, subsequent deaths, and so on. Moreover, to contact people with an explanation of the possible correlations with the onset of cancer could cause unnecessary anxiety, since the research could yield a negative result. Thus, any consent sought would have to be gained on the basis of a less-than-honest explanation. If this is the case, would it not be more acceptable to access the records without seeking consent, and then contact at-risk subjects if the hypotheses were established?

Not everyone would agree that the above arguments are convincing enough to permit the omission of consent to access health records which can contain much personal detail, given by the individual solely for the purposes of obtaining appropriate treatment. In practice, requests of this kind are considered on their merits by individual ethics committees who will investigate whether the omission of consent is justified in each case. There is certainly no automatic right of access to medical records by researchers, and in the future it may be appropriate to document in a person's record specific consent (or refusal of consent) for its use in research.

When research is relatively non-intrusive (e.g. the administration of questionnaires which do not contain highly personal material), verbal consent may be sufficient. However, although verbal consent may be acceptable, adequate information must still be presented to subjects first, and the opportunity offered for them to consider whether they wish to participate. An advantage of written consent forms is that they can be used to specify clearly the nature of the project and the freedom of the subject to withdraw at any stage. Verbal consent can be more coercive of subjects, and may appear to be an 'all-or-nothing' commitment to the project once consent is given.

Procedures

In order to ensure that the guidelines for research ethics are followed in practice, it is essential to institute adequate procedures for protocols to be assessed by properly constituted committees. The composition, functions, and procedures of these committees vary widely from country to country, and there are no international guidelines on this matter. Even the names of such committees are different; for example, in the USA they are called Institutional Review Boards (IRBs), in Britain they are called Research Ethics Committees, in New Zealand they are known simply as Ethics Committees (but their remit includes ethical issues in treatment as well as research). These differences are less significant than other variations, such as the scope of membership, the rules of procedure, and the accountability of the committees reviewing research ethics to other bodies, such as hospital boards or area health boards.

We can identify a number of principles which should ensure that, whatever national variations exist, the interests of research subjects and researchers are protected: the principle of independence and impartiality, the principle of due process, and the principle of accountability.

Independence and impartiality

The best safeguard for the first principle is found in appropriate criteria for membership of the committee. Clearly a committee composed entirely of medical researchers could not be regarded as sufficiently distant from the research community, or sufficiently close to the community at large, to make impartial judgements about such matters as degrees of risk and discomfort, or the adequacy of information and consent procedures. On the other hand, a committee lacking the necessary scientific expertise could never make accurate assessments of either the scientific validity and usefulness of the project or the possible risks entailed. It is therefore essential to have a balanced membership on the committee, representing a wide range of perspectives on research, including the various social or cultural milieux of the research subjects. Particular attention must be paid to minority and other vulnerable groups; and the perspectives of patients who are involved in research concurrently with treatment must be properly represented. It is also important to have other forms of expertise on the committee in addition to the relevant scientific knowledge — notably, expertise in law and in religious or philosophical ethics.

Token 'lay' membership is never sufficient to ensure the proper independence of the committee from the scientific community which it is assessing, since the technical nature of much of the material discussed can easily put the non-scientific members at a psychological disadvantage and may lead to a dominance of decision-making by those with expertise in the research area (Campbell, 1987). The National Standard for such committees in New Zealand seeks to avoid this by requiring that the committee consist of an equal number of lay and health professional/ scientific members, and that the chairperson be elected from the lay members (National Standard for Area Health Board Ethics Committees, 1991). Other devices to avoid bias include requiring the presence of at least two lay members to constitute a quorum and/or requiring that all decisions of the committee be unanimous. Clearly, whatever measures are introduced, they should not have the effect of polarizing the lay and scientific members into two separate camps, nor is it desirable that the lay members feel themselves to be always spokespersons for specific sectional or community interests. The committees that function best are those in which the division between lay and scientific/professional is not noticeable. This can be achieved by procedures which give all members of the committee the assurance that their voice will be heard and their opinion respected.

Due process

The assessment of research protocols is a complex matter which cannot be adequately carried out unless committees have clear methods for dealing with the mass of material presented to them. In order to achieve consistency, each protocol must be subjected to the same scrutiny with regard to scientific validity, ratio of risks to benefits, adequacy of information and consent procedures. Standardized application forms are the first prerequisite for such due process. The range and phrasing of questions on these forms is best defined after some experience of the information which a committee will find relevant in order to reach a decision, but at the very minimum questions should elicit the following information: design of study; qualifications of researchers; source of research subjects and their relationship to the researchers; funding of project, including any payments to subjects, and financial or other advantage to researchers; procedures to be carried out and their attendant risks; methods for monitoring and detecting adverse outcomes; safety procedures; method of obtaining consent; use of results, including safeguarding of confidentiality and communication of results to subjects. All applications should include copies of information sheets, consent forms, and information about compensation arrangements for subjects in the event of any injury.

Due process should protect researchers as well as subjects. This entails providing full information about the membership, constitution, and procedures of the committee, and guidance about appeal procedures in the event of a project being rejected. Researchers should, in the first instance, be given the opportunity to attend the committee in person to explain the justification for their project, before any final rejection. It should also be open to the committee to seek expert advice from outside the committee membership in order to clarify and, if need be, correct their assessment of the acceptability of the project. If the outcome is still a negative one, there should exist some other body (e.g. a national ethics of research committee) to whom reference can be made by either the applicant or the committee in order to get a second opinion. Alternatively, an external assessor can be used in the appeal process. (In New Zealand both options are open to committees or to unsuccessful applicants, since the ethical committee of the Health Research Council has been given that function by statute (Health Research Council Act, 1990). However, this function is a purely advisory one, the final judgement remaining that of the ethical committee of the Health Board in whose area the research will be carried out.) It is a serious matter for researchers if their project is totally blocked because of ethical objections, but if the full procedures described above are followed, then one can be assured that the reasons will be sufficiently grave to justify such a step in order to protect the interests of research subjects. It is their interests which must remain paramount in all medical research.

Accountability

An ethical committee which functions without reference to any other body is always in danger of idiosyncrasy in its judgements, or liable to come under the influence of partisan groups of one kind or another. The accountability of the committee should first be ensured by a declaration that its decisions are taken in accordance with an internationally recognized set of guidelines. Most commonly, normative principles will be derived from the Declaration of Helsinki of the World Medical Association, including its subsequent revisions (see Appendix) or from guidelines issued by the Council of International Organisations for Medical Sciences (CIOMS). In addition, each nation will have its modifications and elaborations, produced by government agencies or professional bodies, or incorporated in statutes.

Another form of accountability is derived from the relationship of the committee to the health authority or organization within which it functions. This relationship is of necessity a subtle one. If the committee is too closely allied to the health care institution or authority, then it may lack the essential independence of judgement and critical role which is its *raison d'être*, but at the same time the committee must be answerable in a democratic fashion to those responsible for the health care of the community, or for the good administration of the health care facility within which the research is carried out. The required blend of independence and accountability can be achieved by a careful system of seeking nominations to the committee, which is recognized as a fair method by both the research community and the public at large, a rotational system of membership to prevent the entrenchment of particular viewpoints or sectional interests, and a system of reporting which allows both the health authorities and the public to monitor the activities of the committee, without allowing either breaches of confidentiality or undue influence on its decision-making.

In the last analysis, the worth of such a thorough system of ethical monitoring of research must be seen in the quality of the research work itself. A system which unduly impedes research and constantly frustrates researchers could never be regarded as ethically justified, since much of the ethical justification of medical care rests on the fact that it is under constant scrutiny and improvement by active and well-designed research into its efficacy. However, since medicine is primarily concerned with the well-being of individuals and of the community as a whole, no research should override the human values which medicine seeks to serve.

The use of animals in medical research

According to the Declaration of Helsinki (1989 revision), 'Biomedical research involving human subjects . . . should be based on adequately performed laboratory and animal experimentation.' Earlier in the same code it is stated that 'the welfare of animals used for research must be respected'.

A number of writers have questioned the ethical justification of such an approach, claiming that the use of animals to check on the safety of products or procedures prior to their experimental use is an infringement of the rights of animals. Such writers would view the phrase 'respect for the welfare of animals' as much too weak, since it allows humans to disregard animal welfare when they regard it as justified for the 'higher' principle of respect for the welfare of humans. This, it is claimed, is merely speciesism, a discrimination as reprehensible as sexism, ageism, or racism. The philosopher Peter Singer introduces his book *Animal Liberation* in the following terms:

> This book is about the tyranny of human over non-human animals. This tyranny has caused today and is still causing an amount of pain and suffering that can only be compared with that which resulted from centuries of tyranny by white humans over black humans (Singer, 1975).

Arguments of this kind depend upon the view that the only relevant ethical issue is the amount of suffering which an animal experiences. It makes no difference, it is asserted, what species the animal belongs to, only how much it suffers. According to the animal rights activist Ingrid Newkirk:

> . . . there is no rational basis for saying that a human being has special rights. A rat is a pig is a dog is a boy. They're all mammals (Newkirk, 1986).

It is obvious that if such a view were to prevail, medical research involving human subjects would become a much more hazardous and painful pursuit, or would have to be radically curtailed. At the present time, no new drug can be introduced for human use until its effects have been fully studied on animals. This frequently uncovers dangerous or even lethal effects which preclude its further development. Similarly, animal experimentation has been necessary to develop and refine surgical techniques, and to further knowledge of physiological and biochemical processes and of anatomical structures. It is frequently claimed by animal rights advocates that much of this research is either unnecessary or irrelevant, because the difference between humans and other animals precludes accurate comparisons, or because computer modelling or the use of tissues rather than whole animals would be an adequate substitute for the testing required. These claims are not accepted by those involved in biomedical research, although it is accepted that the *numbers* of animals used could be reduced, and that some tests used in the past were unnecessarily destructive of experimental animals (e.g. the LD 50 test which required that a dosage of a drug be established which would cause the death of fifty per cent of the experimental animals). Reduction in numbers or types of test, however, is far removed from the total abolition sought by the advocates of animal rights. Such an abolition would, in the judgement of the medical research community, put an end to whole areas of research which could never proceed using only computer modelling, or by experimenting on tissues rather than whole animals.

The nub of the issue, however, is to be found not simply in assertion and counter-assertion about whether animal research is a necessary precursor to research on humans, but in a difference in moral assumptions about the status of non-human animals. If it is true that animals have rights, then all the requirements controlling research on humans would have to be applied equally to the use of animals. This would put animals in the same category as human infants (or other human subjects incapable of giving consent), and so would permit their use only in experiments of direct therapeutic benefit to them or in experiments in which there was minimal risk of any harm. But is it correct to say that non-human animals have rights?

Clearly, many species of animal are capable of suffering, not only in the sense of physical pain, but in terms of psychological distress caused by fear, deprivation, being in an alien environment, or being isolated from members of their own species. But we can assert that humans have a *prima facie* obligation not to inflict such suffering on animals, without recourse to the claim that animals are the possessors of rights. This is evident when we consider whether we would put the same obligation upon animals, either in terms of aggression against their own species, or against members of other species. We see no such obligation because we do not regard non-human animals as moral agents who have such constraints on their behaviour. Predators are not morally reprehensible in the sense that violently aggressive humans are. And, although it is true that 'man is the most destructive by far of all mammals' (Storr, 1970) it is only in humans that such destructiveness is blameworthy.

If only moral agents have rights (and corresponding obligations), what are we to say of human infants or of the severely intellectually handicapped, who are also incapable of fulfilling an active role in moral behaviour? Should we treat them as we would experimental animals? The argument must be different in each case. So far as infants are concerned, we have an overriding obligation to nurture them in order to allow their development as full members of the community of moral agents (see Chapter 5 above). To deny this absolute obligation is to undercut the whole ethical basis of human parenting, of the provision of universal education, and to use the vulnerability of infants as a convenience for those who have power over them. (Similar considerations prohibit the sale of children and the use of child labour, restrictions which even the animal rights activists do not place on our use of animals.) In the case of the intellectually handicapped, their right to absolute protection is based upon the crucial nature of their relationships with their fellow humans. We now know that the potential of these individuals for development and a sense of fulfilment can be realized only when they are given every opportunity to become active and cared for members of the human community. Therefore, we have special obligations to them which far exceed our obligations not to harm non-human animals.

In light of these considerations, we can reject accusations of 'speciesism' as not founded upon rational argument. The basis of racial and sexual discrimination is either that *falsely alleged* differences (e.g. in intelligence or in moral capacity) are used to justify unfair treatment, or that *real but irrelevant* differences (e.g. in appearance or in physical characteristics) are used in a similar way. The differences between humans and other animals are both real and relevant to treating them as being of unequal moral status. Humans alone are capable of that moral agency which commands absolute respect. Humans alone carry the responsibility for determining how the welfare of their own species is to be balanced against the welfare of other living creatures. Only humans must decide when it is right to experiment or to desist from experiment: rats, pigs, dogs, and other mammals depend upon the morality of those decisions.

It is clear from the above argument that denying that non-human animals have rights does not in any way justify the unrestricted use of animals in research. On the contrary, since animals themselves have no voice with which to defend themselves, there are powerful moral obligations upon the human community to protect them from unnecessary harm. This obligation is clearly expressed in both international and national guidelines on the use of animals in research. The fundamental principles are stated in CIOMS *International Guiding Principles for Biomedical Research Involving Animals*:

> Investigators and other personnel should never fail to treat animals as sentient, and should regard their proper care and use and the avoidance or minimisation of discomfort, distress, or pain as ethical imperatives.

Increasingly it is being recognized that the suffering of animals is often overlooked, or regarded as somehow less than that of humans simply because it is expressed differently (see B. Rollins, *The Unheeded Cry*). Thus, the CIOMS guidelines emphasize the need to assume the presence of pain rather than its absence, unless proven: 'Investigators should assume that procedures that would cause pain in human beings cause pain in other vertebrate species'.

Another area of concern is the excessive use of animals in some areas of research. A recent estimate stated that forty million animals are used in one year alone in the USA. There is now an emphasis on the minimum number necessary for the validity of any given experiment, and in every case the number used must be justified by application to an independent ethical committee.

Finally, the infliction of pain or distress on animals as part of an experimental protocol is now regarded as quite unjustifiable, and it is the role of animal ethics committees to ensure that alternative methods of research are devised. All invasive and painful procedures must be carried out with appropriate sedation, analgesics, or total anaesthesia, and if the animal will subsequently suffer severe or chronic pain, distress, discomfort, or disablement that cannot be relieved, it must be painlessly killed. The death of animals is thus regarded as morally acceptable (as it is in their use as food), but not the infliction of suffering.

As with research with human participants, research involving animals is now the subject of regulation worldwide. Properly constituted committees for authorizing and monitoring research should ensure that the inhumane practices of some research with animals, rightly condemned by animal activist groups, will be eliminated from both commercial and scientific research on animals. This will not be enough to satisfy the abolitionists, since animals are not accorded rights by such procedures, and so will continue to be used as mere means to human ends (or, in the case of vetinary research, to benefit other animals). Codes which allow experimentation on animals within specified limits (see Appendix for the full texts of relevant codes) give expression to a 'minimal harm' ethic in relation to our treatment of species other than our own. This is far less than the proponents of animal rights believe to be required, and is of course a much lower standard than those applied to the use of humans in research.

Whether we have got the balance of values right is a matter for each individual to decide, but for a person planning a career in science or medicine, there is really no possibility of opting out of being involved in the manipulation of animals for the purposes of both teaching and research. As medical science has developed to the present time (and for the foreseeable future), it is not possible to subscribe to the ideals of scientifically grounded medical care without accepting that humans must come first in our scale of values. Cruelty of any kind is alien to the spirit of medicine, but equally it makes no sense to a person seeking to protect or restore human health to assert that 'a rat is a pig is a dog is a boy'.

Chapter 7

Medicine and society

Introduction

There is a danger of an excessive individualism in medical ethics, at least in its traditional form. The Hippocratic Oath stresses the responsibility of the doctor for the individual patient, but fails to mention whether the health of the society in which the doctor practises should also be a matter of ethical concern. In similar fashion, the Geneva Declaration (a modernized version of the Oath) states: 'The health of my patient will be my first consideration', but makes no mention of the worldwide problem of the lack of facilities for promoting that health. This emphasis on the individual character of the doctor–patient relationship ignores totally the communal dimension of health care. We all depend upon the capacity of our society to provide adequate health care, and when that provision is shown to be inadequate in any given case, we must each be affected either directly or indirectly. (It is interesting that the Declaration made by medical graduates of the University of Otago, New Zealand, includes a brief reference to the communal dimension. Graduands commit themselves not only to the welfare of patients but also to 'the common weal'. How far the graduating students actually notice the extent of their commitment is another matter!)

The communal dimension of health care ethics is deeper than just the threat posed to each individual by an inadequate health care system. Not only is our own sense of security affected by the possibility that the neglected person could be us or someone close to us; we can also feel a sense of moral outrage, that we live in a society in which the sick or disabled are inadequately cared for, even though those who are neglected are total strangers to us. Health — like education — is not easily regarded simply as a matter of individual preference and purchasing power. The failure to distribute it fairly and adequately raises fundamental questions about the quality of our communal life. The moral issues raised are those of basic human rights and social justice. What is a person entitled to by virtue of his or her simple humanity? What are the obligations which every society has to its members in the sphere of health and welfare?

The United Nations Declaration of Human Rights (1948) includes a description of a right to health and welfare provision:

> Everyone has the right to a standard of living adequate for the health and wellbeing of himself and his family, including food, clothing, housing, medical care and necessary social services (Article 25(1)).

But numerous problems are encountered in seeking to implement this right. The first arises from the problem of constantly increasing possibilities for improved health care provision. The more medical 'successes' we have, the higher the expectations are for what medicine should achieve. Thus, supply constantly fails to meet demand, and the right to health care seems impossible to implement. A second — and more theoretical — problem relates to disagreement about the nature of the 'right' which is claimed, and about the theory of justice which underpins such a right. A third problem will remain, however, even if we can come to some resolution of the first two: How is 'adequate health care' to be defined, and what are the procedures that will ensure that such adequacy is achieved?

The paradox of health care

In 1942, the Beveridge Report was presented to the British government. This formed the basis for the welfare state established by the Labour Government in the immediate post-war era. Beveridge discussed arrangements for health care on the following assumption:

> A comprehensive health service will ensure that for every citizen there is available whatever medical treatment he requires, in whatever form he requires it.

This assumption now seems hopelessly ambitious because we are painfully aware that no country, however wealthy, can possibly afford all the possible treatments which might be beneficial to all its citizens. As medical care has become more effective in providing cures for life threatening conditions, the demands on health services have increased in line with people's enhanced expectations of what should be provided. This 'paradox of health care' has been well described by Maxwell:

> The more infant lives are saved the more serious becomes the threat of handicap. The further life expectancy is extended the greater become the demands on geriatric services and long term facilities for the infirm and

elderly. Each new advance which gives hope to another category of sufferers . . . converts a latent need into an immediate and continuing demand (Maxwell, 1974).

The resolution of this paradox depends upon a willingness to view health care provision in terms of its overall impact upon the health of a population, rather than as a series of individual interventions or responses to demand. Co-ordinated planning of this kind is notoriously difficult to achieve, because of the numerous interests, professional, commercial, and political, which operate in the health field. But an approach can be attempted in terms of the interrelationship of three 'Es' — Efficiency, Effectiveness, and Equity.

The first two of these 'Es' are assessed by health research and implemented by the introduction of adequate resource management. Goals and objectives have to be defined for different aspects of the health service, and ways devised to monitor the extent to which they are being achieved. Thus, it might be decided that major causes of premature death should be reduced by a combination of preventive, health educational, and curative measures. Priority would then be given to the financing of the measures selected, and the plan would be adjusted according to whether or not the desired outcomes are being achieved. Such planning solutions, although useful, depend upon a prior social agreement about which goals and objectives are to be selected out of a vast range of possible goals. Since not all health goals can be achieved, however efficient and effective our interventions become, we have to decide which goals are to be given favoured consideration. Therefore we are faced with the problem of equity. How can we ensure that resources available to health care are allocated fairly? On which theory of justice do we base our judgements of equity in health care provision?

Equity and theories of justice

In one sense, equity is quite simply defined: it is ensured when people are treated in as fair a manner as possible by ignoring irrelevant differences between them, but taking account of relevant differences. For example, it is inequitable to deny people the right to vote (or other basic political rights) simply because of their gender or the colour of their skin. These differences are irrelevant to the issue being considered. On the other hand, it is equitable to deny the vote to those who are severely psychiatrically disturbed, or to persons below a certain age, if it can be shown that these factors are relevant to their capacity to make an informed choice. We have here what is sometimes called the 'formal principle of Justice', which can be stated as: 'treat equals equally and unequals unequally'. This formal principle is of some help in ensuring equity in health care, since it identifies the unfairness of the maldistribution of health care resources, for example, by social class, or by geographical region. However, it leaves unresolved the more difficult issue of deciding which differences *are* relevant in deciding health care priorities. Are some people's health care needs more deserving of attention than others? How are we to determine which?

To try to answer these questions we need to look more carefully at the theoretical debate underlying justice theory. Beauchamp and Walters (1989, p. 33) have described six different principles upon which a theory of distributive justice might be based:

1. To each person an equal share.
2. To each person according to individual need.
3. To each person according to acquisition in a free market.
4. To each person according to individual effort.
5. To each person according to societal contribution.
6. To each person according to merit.

If we consider how these might be applied to health care provision, we can see how some seem more in accordance with fairness than others. A stress on acquisition in a free market (Principle 3), for example, fails to allow for the vulnerability and disadvantage created by illness itself. The chronically ill or permanently disabled are certainly in no position to compete equally with their less disadvantaged fellow citizens. The same objection applies to the principle which rewards effort (Principle 4). This is based on the false assumption that there is a 'level playing field' on which all have an equal capacity to look after their own interests. However, the reality of ill-health is that it removes the possibility of equality of opportunity in a competitive situation. (This is not to deny that individual effort has a worthwhile contribution to make to the maintenance or the restoration of health, but fairness cannot be ensured by using effort as a sole criterion for the allocation of resources.)

A different kind of objection can be levelled against the last two principles. These assume that the health of some individuals is to be more highly valued than that of others, either because they have more to offer to society, or because they are more deserving of consideration and respect because of their personal qualities. There are situations in which we use these principles to distribute benefits. Societal contribution may be recognized by appropriate income levels (though this is rarely the way things actually work in income distribution); and honours and distinctions are frequently used as a mark of excellence of character and achievement. However, to allocate health care according to these principles is to base matters of life and death on our highly fallible judgements of individual or social worth. Health is too vital an aspect of individual well-being for it to be dependent upon such potentially prejudiced judgements. In any case, to disregard a person's health care needs because we regard that person as being of lower value than others, would commit us to a dangerous path of discrimination, in which only the worthy or the socially useful are to be accorded full rights.

We appear to be left, then, with a choice between either an equal distribution (Principle 1) or a distribution according to need (Principle 2). Each has some strong arguments in its favour. When there is a valued and scarce social benefit, an equal and impartial distribution would seem to be the fairest method of dealing with the scarcity. All would suffer equally from the scarcity and benefit equally from the benefits available. Although this appears to promote equality, the effect of equal distribution can often be to increase *inequality*, since the scarcity of resources can have a far greater detrimental effect on some groups than on others. For example, a shortage of primary care facilities in a low-income area has much more serious effects than a similar shortage in more prosperous communities which often have greater resources for self-help. Again, an equal distribution of resources across a range of types of service can have disproportionate effects on some particularly vulnerable groups, such as the intellectually handicapped, the very young, or the elderly, who require a high concentration of health care resources for adequate health care provision.

Thus it seems essential to relate the distribution of resources to some criterion of need. Those with equal needs should get equal shares, but those with greater needs should get greater shares. By using need as a criterion we use equality of *opportunity* or equality of *outcome* as a goal, rather than resting content with equality of distribution. It is the 'need theory' of distributive justice which has had the most influence on health care policy from Beveridge on. It does, however, raise some ferociously difficult practical problems, and these problems of implementation will occupy us for the rest of the chapter.

Arbitrating between needs

An area health board has to make substantial cuts in services in order to balance its budget. A major saving would be obtained by closing down some smaller units in outlying areas and centralizing these services in a major hospital. This is an unpopular move since it causes great inconvenience to these smaller communities. An alternative would be to allow waiting lists for elective surgical operations to lengthen, causing inconvenience and unnecessary disability to a smaller number of people, but at a more serious level.

Such hard choices are a commonplace for health authorities at the present time, and innumerable other examples could be given. What criteria should be used to identify the least undesirable option? (There is no ideal option. Some group must suffer to some degree.)

We begin by recognizing that this decision is not one between individuals as such, but between relative funding of different types of service. This is a dilemma peculiar to countries which have some kind of integrated and nationally funded health service, and which therefore already accept the basic premise that it is a national obligation to provide an adequate level of health care for all citizens. Thus, the debate about justice in health care provision is very different in countries like Britain, New Zealand, or Australia from that in the USA, for example, where this basic premise is still not accepted. Decisions about relative spending between types of service provision can be described as macro-allocation, to distinguish it from micro-allocation — choices between individuals about who should receive a scarce resource (e.g. renal dialysis).

To make macro-allocation decisions we need to combine the three factors of efficiency, effectiveness, and equity referred to above, with the overall aim of maximizing the most efficient and effective form of health care delivery to those whose needs are greatest. Using this formula there seems, at first sight, no escape from the conclusion that services must be increasingly centralized in order to enable them to deliver an effective and lower-cost intervention as equally as possible to a maximum number of people. An under-utilized peripheral service uses up resources which could be put to effective use in a major centre.

Is this a fair conclusion? Why should people be penalized in terms of access to services simply because they live in a rural area? Moreover, the effectiveness of health care services can be compromised if they are too inaccessible and located in larger, more impersonal institutions. A service based in a small community could achieve much earlier interventions for the people of that community, and thus be more cost effective in the long run. These counter-arguments illustrate the uncertainty of decision-making in this area. There are bound to be compromises, and frequently the right balance of types of service and of efficient deployment of services will not be achieved.

So far we have been discussing problems of equitable distribution of services to meet roughly comparable medical needs. The criteria for just distribution become even more difficult to apply when we are attempting to compare widely disparate needs. For example, how are we to determine the relative weightings to be assigned to life-saving as opposed to life-enhancing interventions?

A health authority has to consider two competing claims for its strictly limited funds. The first comes from a group of senior cardiologists and cardio-thoracic surgeons who want to set up a heart transplant unit in the region. They have established that the necessary surgical and nursing skills are already available in a local hospital and that there would be a steady supply of appropriate recipients. The second claim for funds comes from a hospital catering for elderly and terminally ill patients. The wards are in a deplorable state and require extensive upgrading and greatly improved staffing levels. There are reports of neglect of patients, and a number of complaints from relatives about the state of the wards and the poor professional standards of the staff. Both schemes require capital expenditure plus ongoing revenue expenditure, and (given some funding from private sources for the transplant unit) the costs are roughly the same. Which project should the authority support, in the knowledge that due to budgetary restrictions the rejected project is likely to be indefinitely postponed?

This example forces us to consider how we might weigh survival for a few against increased quality of life for a larger group. Attempts have been made to provide a formula for such decisions in terms of Quality Adjusted Life Years (QALYs). A health care intervention is assessed in terms of both the *number* of years of life gained and the *quality of life* during those years of survival. However, although QALYs can be useful when we are considering two or more alternative interventions for the *same* group of people (e.g. cardiac surgery versus medication for people with symptoms of heart disease), they do not provide a moral basis for arbitrating between interventions for *different* groups of people. Let us suppose that (a) the cardiac transplantation would gain for the recipients on average between five and ten years of high quality survival; and (b) the upgrading of the geriatric wards would gain on average three to five years of improved quality of life for the patients on these wards before their deaths. These numbers do not tell us that the heart transplantation is the preferred option for the health authority, unless they are always going to favour those who have longer survival prospects (with the necessary intervention) over those who are closer to death. Such an approach would be morally intolerable since it would create a huge bias in the health service against the old and terminally ill, in favour of those who are younger and can benefit from acute interventions. We would end up with a health care system which was seriously 'ageist'.

What, then, might be a fairer approach? We need to look for some kind of criterion that will allow us to suggest a 'basic decent minimum' in health care provision, and to use this to guide the difficult decisions about allocation between groups of patients with totally different health care needs. To help us in this task we shall consider the following account of justice offered by the philosopher, John Rawls.

Maximizing the minimum

When we contemplate the possibility that a group of elderly people could remain in deplorable conditions indefinitely in order to allow for an initiative saving the life of others, we realize that something fundamental is at stake morally. This was expressed by Kant by the principle that we should never treat people as 'mere means to an end'. However worthy the goal of the heart transplantation programme, a more pressing demand for our attention is the dependency of elderly people for whom the society has already taken responsibility and for whom it has a continuing obligation for adequate care. There is thus a prior obligation to meet their needs adequately, before launching new initiatives in life-saving medicine. Here we may perceive a special place for the value of personal freedom as a human quality, which all societies should seek to both protect and enhance. The less an individual is able to safeguard her own freedom, the more responsibility we have to ensure that there is no abuse of the dependency, and that freedom is fostered as far as possible.

These intuitions about the essential aspects of justice have been incorporated in a celebrated theory of justice formulated by the philosopher John Rawls (1971). According to Rawls, if we were to consider the basic constituents of justice under a 'veil of ignorance' (i.e. when we could not know our particular social situation), we would support two basic principles of justice. The first principle (the Liberty Principle) would require that each person be accorded the maximum amount of equal personal liberty compatible with the same amount for all other persons. This combination is designed to ensure a degree of equalization by social arrangements of those deficits in personal liberty which might be created by the fortuitous circumstances of birth, disability, childhood environment, and so on. Thus, the first principle already has a definite bias toward the weak and disadvantaged in a society. However, Rawls' second principle prevents his theory from being a simplistic egalitarian one, in which no differences between individuals in terms of possession of property or other social goods would be permitted. Rather, Rawls believes that it is just to permit, or even promote, such differences, provided the resultant inequalities enhance the position of the most disadvantaged in society. This 'Difference Principle' once more underlines the need to recognize the plight of those often disregarded by society and afforded inadequate care because they do not have a power base which can actively promote their interests.

To what extent does Rawls' account of justice help in the complex issue of the fair distribution of health care resources? Certainly it prevents any over-simplified emphasis on life-saving at any cost. Clearly a health service which always gives life-saving measures a priority will seriously inhibit the possibility of a fair distribution of those resources which defend the freedom of the disregarded and the underprivileged. An outcome of this in health care provision could be that acute services would use up even more of the budget than they do at present, and services which provide basic care and support at a simple level on a long-term basis (e.g. community-based geriatric services) would lose out badly. This does appear to be the case when a 'free market' is allowed to operate in health care. The health services then most favoured are those which appeal to the members of society with the income to purchase them, while the poor and disadvantaged are more and more dependent on an inadequately funded public service, grudgingly supported by taxation.

On the other hand, the Rawlsian Difference Principle serves as a reminder that we need to pay attention to the overall social and economic impact of health care interventions. A service which allows for a healthy and productive younger group can rebound to the advantage of the more vulnerable groups, if the resources generated by their productivity are then devoted to effective programmes of long-term care. If the imbalance moves too far in favour of funding for the disadvantaged, then (paradoxically) it is the disadvantaged who themselves suffer most in the long run.

It is clear, then, that there are no simple solutions to the issues of priority which have to be confronted in the allocation of resources to health services. Rather, it is a matter of balancing one set of claims against another in a way which keeps the whole system functioning effectively and without gross disadvantage to any one group. This must be the greatest challenge facing the philosophy of health care at the present time, and it can be met only by a continual reappraisal of the fairness of the current arrangements which (Topsy-like) have grown up over the years of dramatic expansion of medical science.

State-funded care versus private practice

The issue of private practice, and the differential access to health care which that creates, is also a subject of ethical debate. There are those who opt for some kind of entitlement theory of justice which corresponds to the principle 'to each according to acquisition in a free market'. We have argued that this disadvantages those who, for no fault of their own, may already be disadvantaged and therefore it is incompatible with the idea of a caring society. Many will agree with this basic stand but argue that a modified mutual health care system according to the principle 'to each according to individual need' is compatible with a limited private sector. In this sector, they argue, those who can provide service over and above what is required of them to serve our mutual need arrangements can contract with those who wish to pay over and above what they already contribute to our mutual system and provide extra health care services. On this basis, the existence of private medical care is thought to be of no threat to a shared-care system which provides according to need (and availability of resources).

The defenders of private practice would go so far as to say that it offers advantages to all to have such a system. They would say that it reduces competition for the limited resources in the public, need-based system, that it gives the professionals greater earning power which reduces pressure on the public system salary structure (and thus on costs), that it provides a carefully costed system which can streamline care in ways that might be copied where appropriate by the public system, and that it provides more choices and greater individual freedom within the society.

In fact, all in the garden is not always that rosy. Where the two systems coexist, there is often a pressure on the professionals concerned to shift a disproportionate amount of time and effort into the highly paid system. There is also pressure not to reduce the waiting lists in the public system because having to wait for care is an incentive to pay for private care. The best one can say is that where the professionals are highly motivated and acting in accordance with the standards of professional practice that we have outlined, there may be no harm in a two-tier system. However, there is great potential for abuse, and definite pressures to devalue one's involvement in public health care. It is to the credit of most professionals working in both that the standards in their public health practice are so high.

Conclusion

Given the complexity of the debate about health care priorities, it is understandable that many doctors feel a sense of hopelessness about this area of medical ethics. What is the use of getting involved in such social or political matters? Isn't it best just to do what one can for one's own patients, within whatever resources are available, and, when it comes to cuts, to 'defend one's own corner' as best one can?

To take up such a position ignores the possibility that a profession can play a prophetic role within the society which authorizes it to practise (Campbell, 1984, ch. 2). Doctors who refuse to see past the immediate illnesses or accidents dealt with by their speciality are depriving society of an important source of insight and critical demand for change. Of course, no one practitioner and no one group of specialists can see the whole picture in health care. However, if sufficient numbers of health professionals are willing to enter the debate about priorities, an impressively wide picture of the crisis areas in health care provision can be gained.

The purpose of this chapter has been to suggest some of the concepts which doctors and other health professionals should use to improve the quality of the debate about justice in health care, a debate which should be everybody's concern, but to which the health care provider can contribute a lot of detailed description of the inequities in the system. We may summarize the basic framework for a just system of health care provision as follows:

1. Justice in health care provision demands that every person be treated fairly, without regard to their social status, gender, ethnic group, or political views.

2. Since illness and accident strike people in arbitrary and unequal ways, the only fair basis for discrimination is the degree of need for health care.

3. When a society has decided that a health care need should be met, all those with that need should be treated equally, without discrimination according to age, gender, place of residence, or alleged merit as a citizen.

4. In trying to put different needs for health care into some order of priority, we should pay particular attention to the disadvantaged in the society, since their liberty to improve their own health is likely to be most severely curtailed.

5. A basic minimum entitlement to health care has to be defined and applied without discrimination to each person in the society. This

minimum should be defined according to what is required to give each person an equal opportunity to exercise his or her personal liberty.

This attempt to ensure justice by equalizing the opportunity to maintain one's own health, reminds us that no one can ensure the health of another. Professionals do not 'give' people health; they make the achievement and maintenance of health a possibility by removing the barriers to it in the lives of individuals. Ivan Illich makes the point about the difference between health and medical intervention succinctly and well in his book, *Limits to Medicine*:

> A world of optimal and widespread health is obviously a world of minimal and only occasional medical intervention (Illich, 1977).

Chapter 8

Ending human lives

Introduction

Human beings have a deep-seated belief that a person's mode of dying is an important part of the totality that is his or her life. This is quite explicit in the practices and beliefs of some ethnic groups, but is present to a certain extent in all human cultures. The moment of passing on from this world is, therefore, a very important point in the totality of a human life. However, advances in medicine have made the determination of the time of a person's death less simple than it used to be. In the past, a doctor would have visited the dying patient during her last illness and then been called to certify that the patient had died. At times, there would have been a sudden death and the doctor would have elicited the story of the events leading to death, then examined the body and tried to diagnose the cause of death. In either case, the cessation of breathing and heartbeat would be taken as definitive signs that death had occurred. This is sometimes, but not always, still the way things happen.

For some people, death is stayed by, or follows, a period of intense medical intervention in the attempt to rescue the patient from a life-threatening injury or illness. This raises questions about when a human being is dead. If we have a human body which is being ventilated on a respirator, but in which there is no sign of brain activity, ought we to regard that person as dead or alive? As soon as we face the responsibility for such choices, a host of other issues are raised. How should we regard a person in permanent coma? When should we cease to persist with life-prolonging treatment? Under what circumstances can patients decline life-saving measures? Should we ever offer a patient euthanasia or active help to die? We now turn to these issues.

The death of a person

Most western countries now accept the brain-death criteria. These criteria involve absence of eye opening, absence of verbal or motor response to pain, and loss of brain stem reflexes (such as pupil responses, corneal reflexes, caloric response to vestibular stimulation, cough reflex, and response to hypercarbia). These indicate not only that the person concerned has no mental or conscious activity but also that there is profound dysfunction at all levels of brain activity. If the human being concerned is totally unresponsive to these tests, and there is good evidence that there is irreversible structural damage to the brain causing that condition, then there is no hope of that human being ever regaining consciousness. We have taken the view that the purpose of medical intervention and life-saving treatment is to benefit the patient (to effect changes in the patient's condition which now or in the future she would regard as worthwhile). It is clear that an individual in the state we are discussing can no longer be benefited by anything that happens to her body. Therefore it seems to follow that we can cease our medical efforts to keep her alive when she is reduced to this state. However, situations are not always as clearcut as the diagnosis of brain death.

> Horace is a twenty-two-year-old student who has been injured in a road accident. It is now three months from his time of injury and Horace is in the state we call 'Persistent Vegetative State' (PVS). He swallows, breathes, absorbs nutrients from his gut, blinks and sometimes his eyes open and rove around in his head without direction or focus. He is being kept alive by a nasogastric tube and occasional courses of antibiotics for chest infections. There are no electrical or clinical signs of activity in his cerebral cortex.

Patients in this state do not have any mental activity, they do not dream, think or experience sensations because they lack the neurological equipment to do so (President's Commission, 1983; Gillett, 1990), i.e. they are cut off from others. They are literally vacant. What is more, those patients in whom the diagnosis is properly made will never recover.

This is quite different from 'Coma vigilante' or 'locked in syndrome' in which the patient's cortex is intact; they experience things around them and understand what is said to them but have lost all voluntary control of motor function (except usually upward movements of the eyes). In the 'locked in' state the EEG is active as in the waking state, indicating active cortical processing of incoming information, and the patient can sometimes establish effective communication with others. Therefore the 'locked in' patient must be regarded as a person who is tragically incapacitated, as distinct from PVS in which it is hard to defend the idea that the person (as distinct from a mere biological human organism) is still there. In fact, often relatives will say something like, 'It's weird, he's not really there any more, is he?' It would therefore seem that we are not morally bound to try and prolong the life of a patient in

PVS because only a biological remnant of a person remains alive, and there is no longer a person who can benefit from our care. This has led certain people to advocate a neocortical definition of death whereby the death of a person (as a person) is said to happen when the cortex is so destroyed that that person will never recover from profound coma such as that seen in PVS (Gillett, 1986; 1987). It seems that we can say that a person's life has ended when that person enters irreversible coma, even though the illusion that he is still alive might persist and indeed be sustained for a while.

Facing death

Cases of PVS make it clear that there are states in which a reasonable person may well not want to be kept alive. But, for most people, death is an unknown to be feared. This means that the caring duties of doctors and other health care workers do not cease when patients reach a point at which pills, potions, and procedures can no longer benefit them.

We need to prepare our patients for the ending of their lives by being honest about what the future holds. Elisabeth Kubler-Ross remarks (1969, p. 29) 'If a doctor can speak freely with his patients about the diagnosis of malignancy without equating it necessarily with impending death, he will do the patient a great service.' There is no worse situation in clinical practice than the terrible web of deceit that is often woven around a dying patient. This is allegedly done for reasons of kindness but, if we were honest, most clinical staff would probably admit that their reluctance to give people bad news is more often the motive. This reluctance is evident in the case of a little boy who was dying of leukemia.

> John's mother and father had always insisted that he should never be told his diagnosis. He was only eight, and they did not think he could cope with the knowledge that he was to die. One weekend it was arranged that John would have a relief stay in the children's hospice where he had often been cared for. On this occasion, he said that he would be all right on his own and that his mother and father could have a little holiday. They delivered him to the nurses at the Hospice and drove off down the drive. After their car had left, John turned to the sister and said, 'Right, this weekend we are going to get a few things straight. I know that I am dying of leukemia, and that Mum and Dad don't want me to know about it, but I have got a whole lot of questions I want to ask'. Needless to say, it was a humbling and enriching experience for all concerned.

It is unpleasant to have to tell a person that soon they are going to die and it leaves one feeling helpless because no more medical magic is available to combat the process that is killing that person. But the honesty required to deal with this challenge is part of a character that addresses itself to the real needs of people and does not seek to avoid them or bury them under mind-dulling medications.

The need for honesty does not mean that we should be stark and brutal in our communications to patients. Honesty and gentleness are congenial companions in terminal care. We should remember that patients need some hope, however slight, to sustain them through terminal illness, and this should never totally be destroyed. However, this does not justify deceit or evasion (Kubler-Ross, 1969, p. 140) which almost always have bad effects.

> Myra presents herself to the surgeon with tests which are almost conclusive of a malignant tumour of the bowel. He talks to her about her symptoms and the tests which had been done, and tells her that there is a cyst or growth of some kind. The possibility of a tumour is raised in the context of a general discussion of the need for operation and possible follow-up care. Myra has her operation which relieves her symptoms but fails to remove all the tumour which is found to have metastasized to her liver. She is told that the operation has gone well, and that the growth was some kind of tumour, but could not be completely removed. She asks and is told that this will need further treatment. The fact that it is cancer, and that she may well not benefit from radiotherapy or chemotherapy, are then discussed a few days later.

Patients in Myra's situation often express profound gratitude for being told the truth in a way that they could gradually digest. When directly asked whether they should have been told more at an earlier stage, they will often say that breaking the news slowly (but within a reasonable time of it being known) enabled them to cope with it much better. This has the added advantage of making sure that the doctor sticks to proven fact rather than acting on partial information. Often a series of conflicting, half-baked or uncertain opinions about what might be going on, given before the evidence is in, can be worse than a policy of restraint and progressive disclosure.

Treating people as reasonable, and encouraging them to make major decisions for themselves, is part of our respect for patients as persons. But most people also need and want support in facing unknown challenges. This implies that we ought to create a climate of care in which terminal illness and the fear of death can be confronted and dealt with: 'It is the one who is beyond medical help who needs as much if not more care than the one who can look forward to another discharge' (Kubler-Ross, 1969, p. 141).

Suicide

Suicide is a traditional dilemma for ethics. Seneca remarked 'the wise man will live as long as he ought, not as long as he can' and 'dying well means escape from the danger of living ill'(1920). However, other philosophers have strongly disagreed. Kant remarks (1963, p. 151):

> . . . suicide is in no circumstances permissible. Humanity in one's own person is inviolable; it is a holy trust; man is master of all else but he must not lay hands upon himself.

Kant's argument shares common ground with the almost universal rejection of suicide by the great world religions. However, we live in an age of secular reason, and thus ethicists must find other grounds if they wish to oppose pro-suicide arguments.

Kant expresses a common intuition when he argues that we treat a human life as in some sense worthless if we are prepared to take it into our own hands to destroy it at the behest of a human will. Thus, there is an impasse in our moral thought. On the one hand, it goes against our intuitions that a rational person should seek to end his life. On the other hand, we find ourselves in agreement with the choice people make in certain desperate situations where the only alternative is to 'live ill'.

The first intuition leads us to conclude that a person cannot be in their right mind to attempt suicide and, on this basis, our laws empower other individuals to prevent them from succeeding. Thus, you do not commit a crime when you commit suicide, but you also do not have a right to do so (because any other person who happens along can stop you). We have some support for this stance from the fact that most people who are rescued will later regret their attempt. Also, it seems, many people who attempt suicide are in a state of mind which, at their best, they would not endorse; they are depressed, hurt, or emotionally unstable (Barraclough et al., 1974). Therefore, our law enables us to respect their more enduring wishes as autonomous rational beings by blocking their (temporary) pseudo-autonomous (because irrational) intentions. We also recognize that a completed suicide is irrevocable; one does not have a chance to reconsider, and we know that often people do think differently about things as a result of hindsight, and having actually experienced the sought-after event. One cannot, of course, actually experience death and reconsider (not, at least, for the purposes of secular clinical ethics), but one can, and indeed many seem to, come close enough to be dissuaded from repeating the experience; 'the "right" to suicide is a "right" desired only temporarily' (Murphy, 1973).

Aside from these things, we realize that a decision to quit life is sensitive to the way life is for the person who makes it, and that this depends a great deal on how we treat such a person. Thus we realize that we all, implicitly, have played a part in the genesis of a suicide and by condoning the rescue are, in effect, asking for a chance to do better. This is probably why the suicide, particularly of a parent, has such a devastating effect on close relatives and family.

However, there remains the point that a person can elect to sacrifice his life for others, or elect not to have it prolonged by medical means. To level against these actions, an absolute stance based on suicide seems illogical because it seems possible that 'some suicide decisions are quite rational, being taken by people with a very clear assessment of their future lives, so that interference is unjustified' (Glover, 1977, p. 180).

> Irene had realized that she was developing the first signs of the cognitive deterioration that had led to her sister's slow and degrading slide into terminal dementia. She had watched her sister lose control over her bladder and bowel, descend from confused speech to animal-like cries and whimpers when her arthritis was plaguing her, and become unable to feed herself or even swallow her food without being tended like a baby. At the end she had been an apathetic remnant of her once vigorous and engaging self. Irene waited for some months until it was clear that the course of her illness was to be the same and then, one afternoon, when her home-help was due, she took a lethal overdose of sleeping tablets. She recorded her reasons and her fears and, when discovered, although she was still faintly breathing, her doctor elected not to intitiate resuscitation.

There is clearly a point beyond which we regard it as immoral and unjust to interfere with the lives of autonomous beings because of our own moral convictions; and it is debatable where this point is reached in dealing with suicide. We shall reconsider suicide in the context of psychiatric ethics (see Chapter 10) but, in general, we seem to have good reasons to intervene in suicide even if this apparently is against the wishes of the victim. In many cases, a suicide is an act of desperation, and our intervention buys time for reconsideration and reconstruction of those things needed to make the individual's life worthwhile.

Euthanasia

The question as to whether we should allow patients to be offered euthanasia raises a number of complex issues. Before we can address them, we need to make certain basic distinctions. *Active euthanasia* involves the doctor killing the patient, and is the only meaning with which we will use the term. Such an action can be at the patient's request — *voluntary* euthanasia — or done without such a request. The latter could involve either a patient who could meaningfully consent but did not do so before her life was ended — *involuntary* euthanasia — or a patient who was incapable of giving meaningful consent to her death — *non-voluntary* euthanasia.

There is also *passive euthanasia*, which involves encompassing the death of another by inaction (declining to perform a life-saving act or withdrawing medical treatment). Because most philosophers do not recognize a moral difference between acts and omissions, they deny the intuitive distinction that many doctors make between killing and letting die. James Rachels' famous case is as follows.

Smith and Jones both have six-year-old nephews and stand to gain if they should die. Both determine to drown their nephews in the bath. Smith sneaks into the bathroom and drowns his nephew. Jones sneaks in with the same intent but before he does anything he sees his nephew slip under the water; he watches him drown.

Rachels asks 'Did either man behave better, from a moral point of view?' (1975). The answer is clearly 'No'. Rachels claims that this shows that there is no moral difference between killing and letting die, but his conclusion seems too strong. One might rather conclude that the difference between killing and letting die cannot rest on whether or not one performs certain active bodily movements.

This means that we have to look further for the reasons for believing in a difference. The British Medical Association gave a number of such reasons in their report on euthanasia (1988, pp. 23-4):

(i) Medical knowledge is limited and it is presumptuous, even arrogant for a doctor to determine the moment a person will die.
(ii) The pressure for active euthanasia can often be met adequately and more creatively by suitable and sympathetic terminal care.
(iii) There is some connection between euthanasia and suicide and most who are rescued from suicide attempts are later very glad to have been.
(iv) There is a danger in making the intent to kill part of our medical ethos.

Their discussion made certain distinctions. The first is between dehumanizing and intrusive treatment solely for the purpose of prolonging life, and 'true' medical care or 'rescue' (this is a bit like the distinction between 'ordinary' and 'extraordinary' treatment).

Alfred is an elderly man with metastatic cancer of the lung. He is
admitted with an acute episode of breathlessness and is found to be
emaciated, anorexic, and exhausted. He claims that he has had enough
and that he does not want any treatment. His wife and daughter remark
that they have expected this for some time, and they agree that he ought
not to have extensive medical tests and treatment. The admitting doctor
notes that he has a swollen left leg, and a chest examination reveals an
area of decreased air entry. She records a diagnosis of deep venous
thrombosis with pulmonary embolus and orders a chest X-ray to
confirm it. She then charts Morphine 10-20mg as required for pain relief
and a nocturnal dose of Amitriptyline. She discusses the management
with the patient and his family and writes a 'Do not resuscitate' order in
Alfred's notes.

This doctor is prepared to let her patient die because there is no available
course of medical management which will rescue him to a satisfactory
state of living. The treatments and tests which might have been arranged
— venography, VQ lung scan, anticoagulants, possible cardio-
pulmonary resuscitation, and so on — are intrusive, costly, and offer
little potential benefit. In such cases, many doctors, having discussed the
situation with the patient and his relatives, may decline to offer certain
medical treatments even though they stand a chance of prolonging life. A
cardio-pulmonary resuscitation, in the circumstances described, is just
such an intervention and would not be indicated because it could not
substantially benefit the patient.

   This, in effect, is a decision to let Alfred die, but it is worlds apart
from acceding to a request to help him to die here and now. The
withholding or withdrawal of medical treatment from someone who
cannot benefit from it does not open the door to medical killing, because
it is based on compassion for the sufferer and wisdom in our use of
medical technology. An active decision to kill or help to die could,
however, be based on motives that vary widely from kindness and the
wish to spare suffering, to a policy of expedient eradication of those who
cannot be helped by medical science. In Germany, for instance, the very
mention of euthanasia provokes howls of public protest. These
considerations require that we give cogent reasons why killing patients
(even with their consent) is not the right thing to do.

   The first is the matter of *intent*. There are, of course, well-intentioned
motives for voluntary euthanasia. The doctor may wish to be kind and
spare his patient terminal distress and agony. He may wish to show his
respect for persons by letting them end their lives at a point where they
are threatened by the possibility of becoming 'infrahuman' with no

remaining dignity or integrity. He may wish to accede to his patients' wishes about their modes of death; after all, if patients are autonomous why should they not make this final choice?

Many doctors would agree with some of these motives. There are, however, a number of ways of serving them. A patient can almost always be given a judicious mix of anxiolytic and analgesic medications (such as Morphine and Amitriptyline) to ensure that he will not suffer even where, with his full knowledge, they may weaken his biological urge to live and so shorten his life. This places a high importance on the *intent* with which a doctor acts. Where the intent is solely to relieve distress, the act can be countenanced by any doctor; but where the intent is to kill, it becomes quite different. In making this point, we are not claiming any special status for medical decisions. There is, in fact, a clear moral and legal distinction between murder and manslaughter, and the crucial difference hinges entirely on the prior malign intent of the murderer. But why do we reason this way in both medical and legal argument?

We can probably trace this reasoning to the settled habits of the heart that form the characters of human beings. For health care workers, such habits are part of the healing ethos. It takes a certain kind of character to detect and respond to the real (sometimes concealed) needs of dying patients. However, in clinical practice, subtle and careful sensitivity to such needs is often diminished where a problem can be solved by purely technical means. Some doctors enjoy such interventions, and therefore avoid the personal and emotive aspects of patient care that are bound to be central in clinical disciplines such as palliative or terminal care, and psychiatry. Active euthanasia is, of course, an intervention to be used when a dying patient's problems become too difficult to cope with. But many hospice doctors volunteer the information that even their patients who are suffering unbearably on admission to hospice care almost never need purely technical interventions, such as increased levels of pain relief. The answer does not lie with 'panalgesia' but with caring human counsel; 'where humane care and a positive affirmation of the value of each person (no matter what their condition) is the prevailing clinical attitude (hospices are a good example) euthanasia requests are rare' (BMA, p. 24). Thus, we are toying with a potentially tragic cocktail when we mix a soupçon of the intent to kill into the attitudes of those who care for the dying. It is too tempting to put an end to difficult problems in clinical practice. Therefore, terminal care doctors, even more than other doctors, must guard their sensitive and caring intuitions.

There are other reasons for this stand. First, there is some evidence that a proportion of people dying from an incurable disease are asking the question 'Am I still worthwhile?'. To answer this question with euthanasia is something about which we ought perhaps to feel reservations.

Second, human death is a very individual thing and medical knowledge is limited. There are unpredictable and unknown aspects to an individual's death which, for many, make their last moments of inestimable worth. It would, therefore, be presumptuous to intervene at such a time with a ready-made technique to absolve us of the need to face this crisis as persons of depth. What is more, because people differ in ways directly relevant to how they end their lives, it is very hard to develop general indications for human euthanasia similar to those we have for animals. When we consider the needs that bring people to hospice care, and the relative unimportance of pure pain relief in that context, this becomes quite evident.

Thirdly, it is unclear to what extent hospice care of the type practised in, say, Britain, is available where there are strong demands for euthanasia. When the alternatives are limited doctors are sometimes forced into desperate measures.

Despite all these worries, active euthanasia by doctors is available to patients in the Netherlands, and seems to answer a very real set of needs. A doctor can administer euthanasia when certain clear conditions have been met and, although he is technically guilty of murder, he will not be prosecuted for it under these conditions (Leenan, 1987). Even there, however, many feel very uneasy about the whole practice. Some of their worries have been discussed already, and similar worries have been voiced by doctors in countries other than the Netherlands.

(i)   Some feel that the fear of death, particularly death from AIDS or cancer, has been exploited by those who advocate euthanasia, and argue that most patients can be managed without this desperate expedient.

(ii)   Some worry that the active termination of life will be extended to cases where the clear conditions of voluntariness and a settled, carefully considered choice do not apply.

(iii)   Some worry that the practice of euthanasia will create pressure on elderly and vulnerable patients to comply, which might affect particularly those individuals most in need of support and care from others.

(iv)   Some fear that if the doctor is seen as being prepared not only to cure but also to kill, the ethos of medical practice and the confidence which patients can have in their doctors will be eroded.

The situation is clearly not as simple as Rachels and others make it out to be. Human death is an unknown, surrounded by fears and uncertainties, and distress of all kinds, and its dynamic is not the kind of thing that is amenable to a model which encourages decisive medical interventions. Thus, we should be cautious about moves to allow doctors to intervene, even at the patient's request, and end the life of that patient.

Quite aside from the particularities of the dying patient, there is a great temptation in modern medicine to develop powerful technologies and efficient interventions which obscure the fact that our patients are increasingly turning to health professionals as persons. When faced with a problem that may seem insoluble, it will often emerge that the real issue concerns communication and relationships. (In fact, a great majority of the ethical problems in contemporary clinical practice have to do with such issues.) Closer attention to the humane art that is medicine, rather than the technical discipline it threatens to become in a cut-and-dried, cost-effective world, would almost certainly avoid many of these problems. One contemplates with horror the kind of society where death and its mysteries are seen as a fleeting problem; where expediency and general contentment are all. Where we have ready answers for all 'sticky' human dilemmas, we seem to end up with a type of human life that is 'sub-human' (which is probably why most people regard *Brave New World* as an anti-Utopia). Therefore, we would argue that compassionate, restrained care and the judicious use of those resources that have a proven beneficial role in terms of pain relief, comfort, and dignity are the best response to the needs of people with tragic and terminal diseases.

Chapter 9

AIDS: poison in the spice of life

Ethical responses to AIDS

The ethical challenges to be faced in our clinical care for patients with AIDS include informed consent, the public health issues, the problem of stigmatization, the clinical relationship, confidentiality, and our medical response to terminal disease. It is the unique clinical profile of HIV/AIDS which forms the basis on which the ethical issues must be discussed.

(i) AIDS is, at present, a fatal disease caused by Human Immunodeficiency Virus (HIV).

(ii) HIV is a virus transmitted in fresh bodily fluids, most commonly during sexual intercourse, particularly anal intercourse, but also through sharing needles in intravenous drug abuse, or through receiving contaminated blood products. It is transmitted to the foetus in thirty to forty per cent of cases involving HIV positive mothers.

(iii) Most cases of HIV infection probably go on to develop AIDS although the rate of progression is variable.

(iv) It is possible that new agents, such as Zidovudine, may influence progression to clinical disease or the course of the disease.

This combination of features, as well as the fact that there exists a vulnerable and already marginalized group in society — active homosexual men — who are the principal victims of AIDS, set the agenda for our ethical discussion.

1. Informed consent and HIV testing

The clinical profile and natural history of AIDS mean that it is quite traumatic for a person to find out that he is infected with HIV. The psychological response to a positive test result varies a great deal (Deuchar, 1984 and Coxon, 1990). Some individuals become severely depressed, even suicidal; some experience a tremendous upsurge of guilt, often associated with feelings of uncleanness; and some cope very well. The typical pattern of shock, guilt, denial, fear, anger, sadness, bargaining, acceptance, and resignation, described by Kubler-Ross for dying patients, is also often seen, in whole or in part, in those who learn they are HIV positive. This is an understandable pattern of response, in that AIDS ranks with cancer as a feared disease. Some patients enter into a state of irresponsible hedonism in which they determine to 'enjoy' their remaining life with an intensity that sometimes borders on the pathological. In others a 'darker' motive appears, and they form the intent to infect others with the 'curse' they see themselves as having fallen under. Yet others become withdrawn, ascetic and severe in their personal relationships. The more extreme reactions may be associated with the extent to which the individual is unhappy with his 'gay identity', but there is no good evidence that this is so.

In any event, it is clear that to learn one is HIV positive is to undergo a change in life. Sexual relationships, which could once have been seen as a pleasurable aspect of life, have to be regarded as potentially hazardous to one's partner. This poses a dilemma to the patient as to whether to be honest and risk sexual rejection, or to be discreet or even deceitful in a close relationship (this is, of course, not so psychologically taxing in a casual/transient relationship). The implications of one's HIV status are often misinterpreted, and the emotional effects can be profound. For this reason, it is important to counsel the patient, and to give realistic information and preparatory advice before the test is taken. There is, in fact, widespread consensus that HIV testing should be the subject of informed consent.

2. Public health issues

Many people argue that HIV testing and the treatment of AIDS are not adequately dealt with under the rubric of autonomy and respect for individual rights because AIDS is a public health menace. This reaction is excessive in the light of the facts about the disease.

The facts about transmission suggest that there is no purpose to be served by mandatory or general HIV testing where the results are to be linked to specific patients and made available for public health purposes. Unlike tuberculosis, which could be caught by casual contact with an infected person because it is primarily a droplet-borne infection, HIV cannot be transmitted in the same way. The fact that direct inoculation by body fluids is necessary to transmit the HIV virus means that the average citizen walking down the street, going into a restaurant, sharing a crowded bus or being served by a shop assistant is at no risk; 'ordinary human intercourse, bar the sexual, is . . . of no risk at all' (Smithurst, 1990). Thus, the hysteria surrounding quarantine, compulsory notification

of particular cases, informing employers or other social contacts, is
both unnecessary and unethical. There are a limited number of relatively
avoidable situations where individuals can be infected by the HIV virus,
and the risk in these situations can be minimized by taking appropriate
measures (such as the use of a condom).

This reinforces a point repeatedly made by Justice Michael Kirby, that
the single most effective public health measure to limit the spread of
AIDS is education and the encouragement of responsible and caring
sexual behaviour (Kirby, 1989). Those most at risk have, in fact, realized
this: 'the homosexual community, which initially had a very low take-up
of testing, has achieved a remarkable slowing of the rate of the spread of
HIV; this has been largely effected through behavioural change'
(Pinching, 1990). The public cannot be protected by attempting to detect
and notify every new case of AIDS, and the ill-informed, 'knee-jerk'
response to the statistics that leads to this kind of measure is only likely to
increase the difficulties in achieving effective control, and perhaps
eradication, of the disease.

HIV testing for epidemiological purposes is, however, clearly an
important (Gillett, 1989) and, indeed, in the light of statistics from New
Zealand and overseas, essential part of a rational response to AIDS
(Skegg, 1989). The obvious worry is that if informed consent is needed
and if, as we know, those who refuse to take the test in an STD clinic
setting are those most likely to have positive results, then the data derived
from a study of HIV status on a sample population will be grossly
inaccurate. This impasse is resolved once it is realized that the need for
consent is based on the fact that important information is discovered
which is identifiable as belonging to a particular patient, and that the
epidemiologist does not want such information. Therefore, as long as the
HIV results are derived in such a way as they are not able to be traced to
individual patients, it can be of no material concern to the patient that the
test has been done. We could even say, providing a special venepuncture
is not performed, that nothing had been done *to that patient* as an
individual at all. Thus, one can justify taking unidentified blood samples
for epidemiological tests of HIV status without the consent of those
whose blood was tested.

3. HIV tests and conflicts between patients

We have suggested that ethical considerations mean that informed
consent is a prerequisite of HIV testing of individuals. This implies that
we cannot force any person who does not wish to to be tested to have an

HIV test. That conclusion is grounded in principles of autonomy and respect for individuals, but there are situations in which more than one individual is concerned. In such situations, the possibility of a conflict of interests suggests that we must pay some regard to the principle of justice. The least troublesome situation concerns blood transfusion. Here, the overall aim is to benefit the recipient of the donated blood. But the patient will be harmed rather than benefited if the blood carries live HIV particles. Therefore, the doctor taking the blood for transfusion purposes has to satisfy herself that the donor is not infected with HIV. This means that HIV testing can reasonably be required on entry into the blood donation programme. It is, of course, a voluntary programme so that the tests which must be performed on participants can be avoided by simply declining to volunteer.

A more difficult problem concerns the procedure to be adopted if there is a needlestick or other penetrating injury in a health care setting. Here, the issues can rapidly be clouded beyond the point of reasonable debate. First, the likelihood of transmission of HIV is slight even when the patient is HIV positive; second, the status of the patient at the time of the injury is not an infallible guide to the risk to the health care worker; third, there are no recorded cases of patients refusing consent to HIV testing under these circumstances; and, finally, it is unwise to form general policies on difficult cases.

The risk to a health care worker from exposure to body fluids from a patient with HIV infection is something between 0.1 and 0.7 per cent (Marcus and the CDC Co-operative Needlestick Surveillance Group, 1988). Thus, most of the time, even if the patient is HIV positive, and there has been a penetrating injury with blood or body fluids, the health care worker has nothing to fear. For this reason, no momentous decisions ought to be based on the result of a test on the patient. However, the possibility that Zidovudine or similar substances may modify the course of the infection makes it important to ascertain whether the injured person is truly at risk. Thus, a case can be made that the injured person has a right to know if the patient whose blood is involved is HIV positive.

However, there is a 'window' between infectivity and positivity on HIV testing, so that even a negative result is not clear proof that no risk exists. The fact that patients, by and large, appreciate the concerns after needlestick injuries, and feel some obligation to those looking after them, implies that Draconian measures designed to license mandatory testing on uncooperative patients are both ill-informed and unnecessary.

It therefore seems that a reasonable policy in this difficult situation would be to inform patients that in the unlikely event of an accident a test for HIV (and other infective agents such as Hepatitis B) would be required, and that they can indicate whether or not they would wish to know the result. If a patient objected to this procedure, an authorization for mandatory testing would be justified on the grounds of a justice — consideration of the interests of all parties concerned. As things stand, it is unclear who could give such authorization. In any event, the recognition that this procedure would be followed would probably obviate any difficulties with unreasonable and uncooperative patients. (The patient is regarded as unreasonable here because of the failure to act out of reasonable or decent consideration for the welfare of others who have provided care, not for any more general reason.)

4. The doctor–patient relationship

Treating AIDS sufferers as a stigmatized and hostile group whom the 'clean' members of society must detect and isolate is exactly the kind of thing that will threaten the balanced three-way relationship between the doctor, the patient, and the community that is required to deal with any health threat. Many doctors imbibe the stereotypes that prevail in upper middle class society, and in the case of AIDS these are potentially disastrous. Doctors and other health care workers who encounter new cases of AIDS need to (and generally do) develop deep commitments to their affected patients, and earn the trust of those groups from which most new cases will come. They cannot do this if they subscribe to damaging stereotypes. The doctor should be aware that a person at risk of AIDS is a potential ally in the fight against a life-threatening disease, but one who may feel very insecure. Often the values and lifestyle choices of the at-risk patient are quite different from those of his doctor and, therefore, he may see the doctor as representing many of the attitudes he has come to feel alienated from through rejection by family or straight friends (Coxon, 1990, p. 149).

The potential problems in the doctor–patient relationship can become serious when a person finds he is HIV positive. As the pressures mount and, perhaps, certain unresolved personal tensions surface, the doctor must be sensitive to the thoughts and feelings that often need to be expressed, even if only so that the patient can work them through in an atmosphere which is not charged with suspicion and fear. A doctor can fulfil the role of counsellor and confidant in this situation and help the patient to find the personal resources to meet the crises he will face. Among these crises are the threats to personal relationships that arise when someone finds that he is HIV positive.

Confidentiality

Terry is tested for HIV after having been on a Caribbean holiday and is found to be positive. In talking to his doctor about the result, Terry agrees that there is a risk to John, his partner, but refuses to allow him to be told. He claims that John will become very jealous and upset, and may walk out on him. He also resists the idea that he should start using condoms because he believes that this will make John suspect that there is something wrong.

The General Medical Council of Britain (GMC) is one of the few professional groups which has addressed the difficult conflict between confidentiality and the duty to warn that is potentially raised by finding that a patient is HIV positive. The GMC stand has recently been followed elsewhere (Statement by NZ Medical Association). If the patient is in an active sexual relationship, whether in a marriage or with a gay partner, there is a real and identifiable risk posed to the sexual partner of the patient. To ignore this risk would be to deny the presumption that, where it is within his power, a doctor will keep another person from harm, whether or not that person is his own patient. (It is on this basis that doctors and nurses stop at the roadside to help at accidents and provide emergency care centres which are not linked to any established health care arrangements or responsibilities.)

It goes without saying that the doctor who has an HIV positive patient ought first to counsel the patient about the meaning of that result, and discuss its implications for his sexual partner. On occasion, this may fail and the doctor may become aware that the partner is being put at risk. What then? The GMC states: 'there are grounds for disclosing that a patient is HIV positive to a third party, without the consent of the patient only where there is a serious and identifiable risk to a specific individual who, if not so informed, would be exposed to infection' (General Medical Council, 1988). But is this advice ethically sound?

We might argue that the magnitude of harm resulting from an uninfected person developing AIDS far outweighs the harm done to the individual whose confidences are breached. This is true and, indeed, is given as a justification for infringing the rights of an individual in other areas of conduct. It is, however, a delicate path to tread. How much, and when, are we entitled to dismantle a traditional aspect of the relationship between doctor or health professional and patient to protect a third person?

We could claim that abandoning a moral constraint is justified whenever one party to the trust is acting unreasonably or in bad faith. This is the basis for revealing confidential information shared by a psychotic patient who does not rightly perceive the consequences and moral import of his intentions, and whose own autonomy or individual rights are suspended until he can again take a responsible place in the society. That is part of the rationale of the decision in the Tarasoff case, where the court judged that a doctor should warn a potential victim on the basis of clinical information obtained from a psychotic patient. In that case, a great deal of discussion turned on the mental disturbance causing the dangerousness of the patient and the view that, because of his mental state, he could not be treated as a normal person would. However, it is clear that the AIDS patient is not mentally impaired and does not lose his right to confidentiality on this count.

We look to be on more promising ground with the concept of 'bad faith', or what one of us has called elsewhere 'moral free-loading' (Gillett, 1988). This occurs whenever an individual behaves in such a way as to undermine the credibility of his appeal to certain principles. The patient who expects confidentiality is appealing to the value that normal and sensitive people attach to the feelings and reactions of others. Because the attitudes of others matter to them, they do not wish those others to be told things which might damage those attitudes. Terry's concern for confidentiality, therefore, arises from his desire to remain in the allegedly caring and supportive relationship he shares with John. But his own disregard for John's welfare, in a sense, undercuts his claim that the relationship is of the valued sort; indeed, it implies that it is far less.

We could compare this with the situation in which parents negate the presumption that they are acting in the best interests of their children by abusing them (i.e. treating the child in such a way that those interests are jeopardized). In this case, we deprive the parents of their normal authority in decisions affecting their children because that authority is based on their claim to be the proper representatives of their children's interests. We reason that the parents' behaviour evinces bad faith, 'moral free-loading' or rational inconsistency with their presumed commitments. By parity of reasoning, we would suspend the HIV positive patient's right to confidentiality because that is based on a presumed sensitivity to and care for the other which is inconsistent with his intention to expose his partner to harm. The unconsented warning is, of course, a last resort and meant to be acted on 'in a fashion that would preserve the privacy of his patient to the fullest extent compatible with the threatened danger' (California Supreme Court, 1976: *Tarasoff* vs *Regents of University of California*). Doctors cannot be ethically obliged to act as accomplices in immoral and dangerous actions.

It is worth noting that the honesty encouraged by the doctor's intervention might well allow a more constructive and co-operative/ caring management of the patient's needs for support and commitment should he develop the full manifestations of AIDS. This 'moral free-loading' argument does not, however, undermine our traditional commitments in any more general way than to devalue those in which the values appealed to are incommensurate with the behaviour shown and evince bad faith on behalf of the one making the moral claim.

A terminal illness

The grim prospects of a patient with AIDS have occasioned renewed interest in the relationship between suicide and euthanasia. Opinions vary greatly on the correct way to respond to these issues. On the one hand, philosophers are prepared to accept that both suicide and euthanasia can be rational individual choices; 'if there is a right to commit suicide, then, arguably, there is a right to competent medical advice as to how to do this, and to information on obtaining the means, and even perhaps to direct assistance' (Almond, 1990). We have discussed these arguments already. It is noticeable, however, that calls for the legalization of euthanasia are more muted from AIDS groups than other quarters, and most commentators have serious reservations about any such move.

The main worry is that a group which is already stigmatized to some extent would be particularly vulnerable to the drive whereby an awkward situation was dealt with quietly and conveniently rather than by careful consideration of the deep ethical and personal issues involved. If the normal patient is vulnerable because of the medicalization of death, how much more the patient who is already seen as being slightly marginal. If a young person with all sorts of difficulties coming to terms with his or her life and identity is liable to make rash and tragic decisions, how much more is a person who feels guilty and is perhaps struggling with emotional problems because of sexual identity, lifestyle and, perhaps, estrangement from his family. All these factors make the AIDS patient more likely to be vulnerable to the tragic counsel of a gentle (but not necessarily fitting) death. One's own wishes in this regard are likely to be uncertain and unsettled, as the widely varying reactions to an HIV test result show. It therefore seems that there are special reasons to worry about euthanasia for AIDS.

We have so far said little about the ethical impact of drugs to treat AIDS. If Zidovudine/AZT, or other drugs like it, come to offer a reasonable prospect of cure or control of the virus, then some of our problems will lessen and others intensify. We will have to consider the problem of a life-saving treatment whose availability is limited by expense and opportunity, and deal with the potential problems created by a black-market operated by entrepreneurial 'patients'. On the other hand, HIV will no longer be directly linked with death, and therefore some of the emotive and fearful hysteria attached to the disease will be removed. AIDS will occupy the spot once occupied by syphilis, and we will have to reconsider the ethics of detection, notification, and contact tracing, because issues of individual patient welfare and public welfare will become congruent; it will be in everybody's best interests to detect those who are HIV positive. We will also have further cause to examine the disparity in treatments available to the rich and the poor in those countries where health care is recognized as a public good only in a very attenuated way.

The production of treatments for AIDS/HIV should cause us to reflect on the ways in which doom-criers and flag-wavers produce an overreaction to a historically limited phenomenon. It should, therefore, warn us about the advisability of legislation relating to drastic measures such as euthanasia for a disease in which the therapeutic possibilities are in evolution.

The challenge to the health care professions implicit in the unique profile of AIDS fundamentally concerns their role in dispelling the myths and stigmata that attach to the disease.

> AIDS victims have been fired from their jobs, driven from their homes by terrified and ashamed families, and abandoned by similarly disposed lovers. The body of one patient was disowned by his family, and funeral directors are declining to handle the bodies of others (Deuchar, 1984).

The near-hysteria found in some circles cries out to be met by reasoned ethical discussion which recognizes the issues and examines them in an analytic but concerned manner. This is a charge on the health care professions, and a responsibility they ought to accept in accordance with their duties to individuals and communities that look to them for expert help and guidance.

AIDS also presents a challenge to our legislative morality as a caring society. Legislation too often reflects the cynical morality of vote-catching, rather than a considered response to a crisis needing careful, compassionate thought. Vote-catching by subscribing to slogans and stereotypes and feeding off public anxiety is a notorious tool in the political armamentarium. Unfortunately, these are incompatible with a well-ordered set of policies designed to preserve a caring and decent society. We certainly cannot claim that we have a caring society when a minority that risks being marginalized is excluded from our community of care, and made the target of public fear and insecurity. This has happened all too often in history and with well-known results. It is to be hoped that it will not happen again in the case of AIDS.

Chapter 10

Mad, bad, sad, or glad?

Introduction

Psychiatry and the disorders that it encounters pose special ethical problems which are not quite the same as those in other areas of medicine. However, the basic approach we have outlined, and the principles that it yields, are quite applicable to this unique area of discussion where, for instance, an autonomy-based account has some almost intractable problems.

Patients with psychiatric disorders suffer, in one way or another, from an impairment of the mental and moral faculties that underpin our lives as ethical creatures. The patient's autonomy — his ability to make reasonable decisions about his own preferences and interests — rests on just these faculties and is the basis of the medical partnership. Because a psychiatric patient's actions do not fit the normal pattern of personality function and the self-regarding interests that constitute autonomy, we cannot treat him as we would a 'normal' person who may have an impairment of bodily function but whose thoughts and emotions remain more or less intact. The fact that psychiatric illness affects the character, thoughts, and feelings of the patient, makes us unsure whether a person's wishes about treatment can have the same pivotal role that they are given in other clinical situations.

These facts raise ethical problems about psychiatric diagnosis and classification, the nature of the doctor–patient relationship, compulsory treatment, psychosurgery, confidentiality, suicide and its management, and reproductive ethics for psychiatric patients.

Diagnosis, classification, and stigmatization

A diagnosis that one is psychiatrically disordered classifies a person as abnormal in a very fundamental way. To some extent, a person's physical condition is able to be defined quite separately from any comment on the kind of person he is. But a judgement that one is disordered in the mind is not so easily separable from the gamut of personal and moral attitudes that others take towards oneself. Thus, psychiatric patients are often stigmatized as being somehow tainted in the essence of their identity as persons, and not just as afflicted by an incidental condition. They are called names: 'loonies' (touched by the moon), 'nutcases' (something wrong in the head/'nut'), 'mentals' (something wrong with the mind), or 'crazies' (unpredictable, dangerous). They are also marginalized, set apart as *defective persons* from the rest of society who are 'normal', and this attitude toward psychiatric patients and past patients creates a deep ethical problem for a caring society. There is a legitimate need to take extraordinary measures in order to benefit such a patient, yet the patient himself may resent being classified as disordered in this way and may not see any need for treatment. Therefore, to intervene and benefit such a patient is to treat him as less than a person with regard to decisions central to his life and well-being. Thus, the problem of classification and diagnosis is loaded with ethical significance.

> The roots are primitive, powerful, and universal. When we want to do unto others as we would not have them do unto ourselves, we find some way of turning them into *others*. We usually do that by labelling them, by excluding them from our own group, and by dehumanizing them (Reich, 1981).

The fact that we regard psychiatric patients as radically *other* is based on the fact that they must be treated differently from other people, but also legitimizes treatment which a doctor would never dream of inflicting on others. This means that such patients are vulnerable to treatments which are not directly connected to the desire to benefit them, and may in fact be harmful or degrading. Literature is replete with examples of books written about discriminatory and dehumanizing attitudes masquerading as care of the insane (*Faces in the Water, One Flew over the Cuckoo's Nest, Skallagriig*). In each story, the same processes tend to occur: the patient is diagnosed as mentally disordered, he is admitted to an institution, he is treated as less than a person, he objects to that treatment, his objection is regarded as further evidence that he is unable to see what is for his own good, harsher measures are instituted to overcome his resistance to treatment, 'treatments' are used which may damage him further, he is truly dehumanized — in his person, not just in his *persona*, the defects of relationship and conduct that existed at the outset are amplified and fixed so that rehabilitation becomes a more and more remote possibility.

The problems do not start with the process that follows the making of a psychiatric diagnosis. They begin within the diagnostic event itself and even, in some cases, long before it. Writers such as Laing (1965) and Szasz

(1983) have critiqued psychiatric diagnosis as a process of evaluation of the conduct of those whom a society (or micro-society such as a family) finds disturbing. Whatever one may think of anti-psychiatry, it has made us take careful note of the fact that psychiatric disorders are not only *intrapersonal* but also *interpersonal*. Most psychiatric diagnoses, even where we are persuaded that a disease model is both realistic and compelling, involve a breakdown of interpersonal relationships, and therefore render the patient vulnerable and needy in him or herself at the very point where help can often be found to cope with the stress of a major crisis in one's life and well-being. Because of this vulnerability, there are special hazards in the therapeutic relationships of psychiatric health care.

Doctors, patients, and therapeutic relationships

The fact that psychiatric illness affects the psyche, implies that the threat to the dignity and self-sovereignty of the patient in psychiatric therapy is much greater than in normal clinical care. The theory that there are unconscious and irrational determinants of the attitudes, interests, desires, and beliefs of the psychologically disturbed person intensifies this 'insufficient regard for the patient's intentionality or will' even more. A *sine qua non* of therapy is to overcome whatever is distorting one's perception and action, and thus the therapist as a person is a key figure. The patient is likely to make normalizing reference to the therapist by trying to reorder her perception of herself in terms of the words and reactions of the therapist. Thus, the therapist's ideas have normative force in shaping the personality readjustment of the patient and her view of what normal interpersonal life ought to be like. The very nature of the relationship means that the therapist's ideas are of paramount structural importance in the psychiatric process. Their structural importance rests in the structure of the relationship where the therapist has the role of discoverer, conceptualizer, judge, and correcter of the patient's problems, and thus the patient is put in a role which can hardly help but be dependent, deferential and, to some extent, worshipful (the therapist must seem to be worthy of respect and admiration).

The individual therapist may be in a position of power which is open to abuse, but the same role can be taken by a group of people. When the therapeutic medium is a group, the risk of individual therapeutic idiosyncrasy is lessened but it is replaced by a no-less-powerful (though more ill-formed) group influence which may be harder for the patient to question, or understand and deal with. If we believe that balanced reflection about and understanding of oneself as a person are important in overcoming a psychological disorder, then these inherent problems of power must be faced and a pattern of practice sketched in which abuses arising from them can be minimized.

In general, there are some clear guidelines to ethical practice in any area of medicine:

(i)   The methods used must be attested and validated as likely to benefit the patient, i.e. tend to return the patient to proper functioning as a responsible and self-directed individual.

(ii)   The professional will always preserve a certain 'distance' from her patient so as to act in accordance with good clinical practice and not on the basis of emotional entanglement.

(iii)   The clinician will refrain from harming or damaging the patient by her advice or actions.

These cornerstones of care can guard a practitioner against some of the worst breaches of professional conduct within psychiatry. The problems may involve emotional or sexual abuse of patients, affronts to the patient's dignity or autonomy, or ill-considered 'treatments' which are not only not proven to benefit but carry uncharted risks of harm.

In part, the problems in psychiatric practice and its regulation stem from the vast array of different methodologies and theories about mental illness. The methodological diversity, in particular, is staggering and therapies like, 'feeling therapy', 'sleep/coma therapy', 'nude therapy', 'screaming cure', and 'orgasm cure' seem vulnerable to abuse by patient and therapist (Karasu, 1981). The breadth and diversity of approaches to, and formulations of, psychiatric disorder make ethical principles difficult to apply to many therapeutic situations. The vulnerability of psychiatric therapy to abuse is compounded by the emotional vulnerability and proneness to exploitation of many psychiatric patients. Patients presenting for psychiatric help may well have been damaged by interpersonal and social injuries. They enter into a clinical relationship which is necessarily 'private, highly personal, and sometimes intensely emotional' (Karasu, 1981). Some patients will look to manipulate the relationship to create an illusion of involvement which is not properly part of professional care, and some therapists will find within a succession of relationships with dependent and adoring patients a source of satisfaction and self-esteem that their non-professional lives may not offer.

The most obvious and widely publicized type of professional misconduct involves sexual entanglement with clients or patients.

Dr H is seeing Dave, a bank manager, for temper tantrums at home and loss of motivation at work. It emerges that Dave, despite an aura of easy-going competence at his job and a very congenial and confident manner with his peers, is actually quite insecure. His lack of motivation at work is related to a fear that he will lose his job, and an inability to complete reports, etc. in case they do not match up to what he perceives to be the high standards required for success. He is also being distracted by what he sees as a passionate involvement with one of the secretaries in the bank, herself a recent casualty of a relationship breakup. His violence at home is related to an increasing intolerance of any indication that he is less than a fully adequate male. Little things such as minor repairs on the car or around the house, or any suggestion of financial constraints on family activities, annoy him intensely and lead to sullen, withdrawn moods in which any family member who crosses his path will be chastised for a real or imagined fault. Dr H begins to work with Dave's sense of self-esteem and do some basic assertion training.

Things at work start to improve but problems at home do not, and Dr H arranges to see Dave and his wife, Elaine, together. These sessions are slightly strained, and Elaine asks for some time in counselling by herself.

Elaine expresses her fears that Dave is having an affair, and also her worries that the recent deterioration in their relationship might have been based on her reluctance as a sexual partner. She mentions that Dave does not seem very interested any more. Her fears about him having an affair are confirmed by Dr H. She says it must be because she is no longer attractive. She is reassured by Dr H. One thing leads to another over the next few weeks, and she and Dr H develop a sexual liaison. When all these goings on come to light there is a major scandal and Dave initiates a malpractice suit.

The complications of this case not only indicate considerable lack of wisdom in Dr H's conduct but also raise the general problem of defining the bounds of acceptable patient contact in psychotherapy. What if Dr H had not had a sexual relationship with Elaine but had merely conveyed to her, by physical and emotive contact, that she was attractive and could regain Dave's attention from his temporary emotional refuge with the woman at work?

> Is sexual contact between therapist and patient unequivocally unethical regardless of outcome? If it is unethical, what about 'non-erotic' kissing, hugging, and touching, that more than 50 per cent of psychiatrists engage in with patients? (Karasu, 1981)

We must surely ask of such practices, admitting our uncertainty about their validity, whether they preserve 'professional distance' and avoid any harm or damage to the patient (as per Hippocrates). On any view of human relationships, it seems quite unlikely that a temporary sexual liaison with a therapist is likely to leave a person more integrated, balanced, less exploited, and more sexually at peace with themselves than they were before that entanglement. Many patients are vulnerable and have a history of unsatisfactory emotional involvements that readily combine to form a witches' brew of psychological forces when combined with exploitation by a therapist. The sexual relationships that are developed in therapy seem to be just that: 'such ostensibly therapeutic sexual interaction almost always involves a male therapist and a young female patient . . . there is little evidence of the rapist providing such help for the fat or ugly who might receive from it more benefit to their self-esteem' (Bancroft, 1981). This astute comment alerts us to the implicit double standards that attach to the kind of rationalizations that are brought to bear on sexual misconduct by professionals. It emphasizes something we tend to forget: that properly validated professional care is a skill to be exercised with care for, but not emotional entanglement with, a patient.

The problem of harm also seems to attend interventions such as aversion, shame therapy, and 'strategic' therapies which demean or humiliate the patient. No doubt there are contexts within which such practices can be used in a restorative, healing way but the intuitive sense that someone is being harmed by being so treated should be closely heeded, and only set aside where clear indications of benefit are well grounded in reputable clinical literature.

A particularly insidious, widespread, and elusive problem in our general care of patients with psychological disorders is the indiscriminate use of drugs where drug therapy is not proven to be innocuous in its effects. In fact, the pervasiveness of this failure of adequate professional care is evident in the medicalizing of life's problems by the use of psychotropic drugs. Many patients have personal and social problems that need positive constructive answers, which may or may not be able to be arrived at by someone working in the traditional medical model. This is just as legitimate a demand upon our expertise as health care professionals as is any other cause of human suffering which presents itself to us. We cannot pretend that we are exercising competent professional care if such problems are met with a speedily scribbled note for some drug and a cursory interview which carefully skirts the patient's real needs.

These types of aberration in care seem quite different, and some at least are hard to detect and correct. We have argued that the validation of clinical skills enabling an informed response to the patient's needs, professional distance, the proper exercise of those skills, and an acute sense of the vulnerability of the patient to the harms caused by psychological abuse, exploitation or depersonalization can go a long way to addressing these problems, and can safeguard mental health professionals from error.

The uncertainties and difficulties of the complex relationship between psychiatric professional and patient mean that professional judgement and wisdom are at a high premium. The vulnerability of the patient puts tremendous ethical weight on the clinical decisions which are made. This is nowhere more evident than in the process of securing involuntary treatment for those we consider to be insane or mentally disordered. These patients not only find themselves suffering great distress but also 'may suffer other indignities or punishments in addition to their liberty being curtailed' (Szasz, 1983). The indignities include enforced medication, which may have unpleasant or serious side-effects, the imposition of a special status for the purposes of employment and other civil entitlements, the administration of the patient's affairs by others, and even being submitted to invasive and potentially damaging physical treatments to attempt to alleviate the problem. The alienating nature of these measures, and the background context of an area of health care in which compulsory treatment is a possibility, have potentially devastating effects on the therapeutic relationship as normally understood which go beyond the interpersonal problems we have already discussed.

Compulsory treatment

The possibility that a close friend, or even oneself, might be forcibly restrained and treated by methods which to many would seem barbaric — such as intramuscular injections, electroconvulsive therapy, or isolation — is truly frightening to most people. The fact that it is done to some members of our community seems to contradict many of the emphases of this book. Compulsory treatment 'is, in itself, an evil; it can only be justified by large countervailing gains' (Hare, 1981). Compulsory treatment is, of course, required only where the patient will not co-operate with efforts to treat his problem. As an institution, compulsory treatment contravenes the requirement to seek informed consent to medical interventions which is part of a therapeutic relationship with any reasonable person. The psychiatrist, in fact, has an unenviable task. She must pay heed to the overriding value of *beneficence* or the desire to help the patient in the face of the patient's (often very suasive) appeal not to be treated. The only way to override the interpersonal appeal of the patient in this circumstance, and yet keep a firm hold on the ethical principles we have enunciated, is to realize that the patient has 'a mental defect which seriously impairs their judgement' (McGarry and Chodoff, 1981). In fact this 'mental defect', along with the considered opinion that the patient may well act to the detriment of his own or others' welfare, are both legally required aspects of the justification of compulsory treatment in most jurisdictions.

The mental defect entails that one of the foundations of our ethical framework is absent, in that the patient concerned is not thinking and acting as a rational social being would. The opinion that this is so and that there is also a real danger to the patient or others is, of course, a difficult clinical judgement to make and, for that reason, should be made, wherever possible, by a clinician with adequate psychiatric expertise. In most countries, this is not a firm requirement and, in the absence of a system which ensures careful review of the decisions made and the right of the patient to appeal, this can lead to abuse.

The institution of compulsory treatment can be softened somewhat by giving the patient information and co-operation where possible. This avoids the 'prisoner syndrome' whereby the patient's often paranoid fears are in fact realized.

> Albert began talking to his landlady about the fact that people were treating him strangely, and expressed the fear that they were going to lock him up. This became a preoccupation, and he began to tell people that the word was getting around and that the doctors were starting to take an interest so that he would not be surprised if one day they did not visit him, take him away and try to alter his mind with poisonous drugs without telling him what they were doing. This all duly happened, and was justified on the basis that Albert was confused and suffered paranoid delusions, such that he did not really understand what was happening to him and he was a danger to himself. The magistrate making out the order for his committal was, not unsurprisingly, a little difficult to convince.

The idea that the patient should be communicated with, and not cut off from developing an understanding of his problems and the strategies which might be used to counteract them, is becoming more and more the norm in psychiatry. It is important that a patient not be kept in ignorance where that can be avoided (even though the patient may not respond appropriately to the attempt at communication) because a key factor in continuing psychiatric treatment is going to be the therapeutic relationships that the patient forms. These relationships aim to restore the patient to autonomous function as a person — a rational, social being. Nothing could be more damaging to such a relationship than the perception that the psychiatrist is an enemy or repressive authority whose mode of action is to confine, disempower, and override the patient as a person.

Attempts to communicate with and include the patient in decisions (which may involve an element of beneficent coercion) enhance the possibility of safeguarding the dignity of the patient in what is necessarily a humiliating situation. When the phase of restoration to something like normal function is reached, the patient must rebuild his personality and relationships on whatever shreds of personal dignity and integrity he has left, and his ally in this process should be the therapist. It is therefore intrinsic to good practice, even where that does involve compulsory treatment, that all that can be done has been done to preserve the semblance of a normal clinical relationship between health care worker and patient.

Psychosurgery and ECT

Psychosurgery began with an operation on the frontal lobes by the Portuguese neurologist Egas Moniz and his surgical colleague Almeida Lima. The standard procedure involved cutting the major connexions, or some large proportion of them, between the frontal lobe — the seat of personality, higher order motivations, and socialization — and the rest of the brain. The effects of the operation are difficult to assess. It undoubtedly helped a number of severely depressed and disturbed patients at a time when little else was available. The state to which many of these patients had been reduced should warn us against making wild claims about the damage produced by the operation itself. However, the operation seems to have flattened affect, impoverished personality and character, and produced a state of motivational destitution that many would regard as inhuman. We must therefore count it as inflicting a serious and irreversible harm as the cost of relief from an identifiable psychological disorder.

Between 1942 and 1954, 10,365 patients were treated by this procedure in England alone. To many contemporary commentators this seems almost incomprehensible, but we ought to recall that little else was available to help those patients at that time.

A further procedure is amygdalotomy which is used to treat aggressive disorders and some types of hyperactivity. Its use is limited to certain geographical *loci*, and in some it has been suggested as a means of controlling violent criminals. The effects of this are relatively uncharted but seem to include motivational alteration. Both procedures carry a risk of death or permanent alteration of psychological function, and, *ex hypothesi*, are being offered to individuals suffering psychological impairments. These features mean that ethical justification is hard to find and, in the face of nothing more than anecdotal evidence of benefit not conferred by less intrusive treatments, may be impossible to defend. The issues should not, however, be obscured by a shock/horror reaction at the very thought of such things.

Similar shock and horror is often evoked by reports of electroconvulsive therapy (ECT), which undeniably did and still does help certain patients. ECT involves passing an electric current through the brain at a level which, unmodified by anticonvulsant and anaesthetic medication, would cause an epileptic fit. It is claimed that ECT has a dramatic effect on certain patients with severe depression, and that it causes no demonstrable harm if administered properly. We cannot hope to evaluate these claims, but we can outline the ethical principles that go into their assessment.

In both cases, procedures are performed which are not well founded on any scientific understanding of psychological function or psychiatric disorders. In both cases, the reason for the popularity of the procedures was that they served to alleviate, to some extent, the intense suffering of individuals condemned to live in great distress, and often with no hope of release from an institution. There is no doubt that the unclarity of the breadth of indications for the procedures, and the desperation of doctors and patients, led to unwise and overly extensive use of both techniques and a failure to soberly consider their possible risks to personality and brain function in the long term. In both cases, there was also serious risk to brain function and a risk of death. Both treatments have been the subject of intensive lobbying by patients and human rights groups, and have drawn the ire of ethicists because of their use without informed consent. None of these facts give us adequate reason to dismiss the treatments as ethically unacceptable.

We must recall that the treatments were genuinely thought to offer hope to those who had no hope and that, on this basis, they passed the test of beneficence on which we have defended compulsory treatment of other types. That is why a treatment which is dangerous, in which informed consent may not be possible, and which may not be proven to produce a benefit, but which is the only alternative to an unacceptable future for the patient, can be ethically permitted. Under these circumstances, a reasonable person might well, in spite of all the drawbacks, opt for a slim chance of benefit. If we would allow a reasonable and autonomous patient to make this choice, it seems perverse to deny a mentally impaired patient the same opportunity. Of course, we would want to know that the medical evidence really did suggest that the choice was reasonable, and the alternatives truly bleak for the unfortunate person, but given those things, it would be not only permissible but even, to some extent, obligatory to offer the patient the chance of improvement. The need to take account of objective considerations, and not merely patients' choices, in assessing these treatments would also suggest that consent to psychosurgery, though the norm where possible, would not be a sufficient justification for undertaking such operations (Kleinig, 1985). Desperate and possibly incompetent patients may well make ill-judged choices, and they should not be exposed to harm through those choices.

Confidentiality

Some psychiatric patients pose dangers to other people, yet do not pose such an obvious danger that they can be committed to safe care. Just such a case led to the controversial 'Tarasoff' decision in 1974 (California Supreme Court, 1976).

> A young male student, P, who had been in treatment for violent tendencies and paranoid ideas, told his therapist that he intended to kill a female student whom he did not name but who could be identified as T from information he gave about her. The campus police were notified, but T's family were not warned. P was detained by the campus police and then released because they thought he was rational. T arrived back from her vacation and P killed her. The family sued the University and the therapists for failure to take proper action which, they claimed, included warning them of the threat to their daughter. The court found in their favour, although it recognized the difficulty of the duty it thereby endorsed, and the conflict between that duty and the duty of confidentiality that forms part of the ethical code for medical practice.

This decision predated guidelines about AIDS/HIV infection, potentially dangerous drivers, and children at risk of abuse. Various bodies have decided in these situations that the magnitude of the harm consequent on an absolute respect for confidentiality outweighs the harm from breach of confidentiality.

We should note that there is also a suspension of the normal terms of the doctor–patient relationship in the compulsory treatment of the insane. Thus, whatever we decide about the aptness or otherwise of the findings concerning professional judgement of dangerousness, and duty to warn in the Tarasoff case, certain ethical principles emerge. Where the therapist becomes aware that any patient has disclosed information which gives her reason to believe that an identifiable person is at significant risk of harm, she should take any measures she can to protect that person. If this involves suspending her normal duty to respect confidentiality, then so be it. This advice embeds a similar standard and set of considerations to the advice given about HIV infection and would, we expect, receive similar endorsement from responsible professional bodies.

Suicide

We have already discussed suicide in general, but we will now reconsider the issues it raises in the context of psychiatric care.

The accepted practice of the medical profession in relation to suicide has been to take whatever steps are necessary to prevent a suicide attempt from succeeding. This is not just because suicide offends our sense of the sanctity of life (and we have argued that seems to be a misreading of the values on which most people make health care decisions) but seems rather to have to do with the finality of death, and the realization that a person must be desperate before she attempts to commit suicide. Taken together, these things lead us to doubt whether the decision to take one's own life is generally well-reasoned, a doubt which becomes even greater when we notice the consistent correlation between suicide and psychiatric illness. However, 'the possibility of suicide is considered by almost every human being at some stage of his life' (Heyd and Bloch, 1981) despite the fact that most of us turn away from that step. Thus, our ethical attitudes in this area are bound to be mixed, and we cannot treat a suicide patient as insane merely because she attempts to commit suicide. There is, however, a gamut of cases ranging from those in which the concurrence of suicidal ideation and major psychiatric disorder make our path clear, to those where it is hard to dispute the (reasonable) choices made.

> Mark has a diagnosis of bipolar illness predominantly depressive in type. He is initially well maintained on Lithium but when seen in the clinic is noted to have delusional and suicidal ideation. He is extremely difficult to engage in conversation and keeps talking about a black incubus sucking his life force out of his brain. He is advised to come into hospital but refuses, claiming that the hospital will suffocate him because of the malignant gases escaping from the cancer ward. His therapist speaks to his sister, and then arranges for Mark to be committed for compulsory treatment.
>
> Heather is a 23-year-old who lives in a city flat with three others. She has recently lost her job as a teacher because of a reduction of the roll at her

school, and now does relieving work in local schools. She presents to the psychiatric service, having been referred for depression. Her parents are separated and living in different cities from her. She has few local friends. She visits the town where she spent her childhood during most of her holidays but, increasingly, finds fewer and fewer of her old friends there. She expresses little interest in the future, and has no pastimes or plans about which she is enthusiastic. Outpatient care, counselling, and anti-depressant medication are all of little help to her and, after attending the service for some weeks and having had an inpatient stay of ten days, she says to her therapist she is going to kill herself. She does not seem mentally impaired and, although the therapist is worried about her, he does not feel he can commit her for compulsory treatment. The police notify the clinic the next morning to say she has been found dead and they are seeking information for the coroner.

Edna and Arthur are a well regarded couple who, in retirement, have enjoyed good health and continued to maintain their contacts with the academic life of the university where he taught for some years. Arthur begins to notice a failing of his memory and general intellect, and a disturbing change of his personality after his seventy-sixth birthday. He recognizes in himself the first symptoms of a distressing form of senile dementia to which his family is prone. Two months after this realization, he and Edna also find out that Edna has a malignant bowel cancer that has spread to her liver, and which is causing her significant and unremitting pain. They plan and hold a party for their many friends and family over the weekend of Edna's seventy-fourth birthday. Three days later they are found dead in their bed from massive overdoses of her analgesic and cardiac medications.

The undeniable link between suicide and mental disorder means that the last of these three cases is not at all typical. However, it does not mean that one can never rationally choose to end one's own life and we have now described two cases ('Irene' and 'Edna and Arthur') where that is not so. However, the fact that a number of those who attempt suicide are making their choice while disturbed, and will not choose that way again, justifies our intervention. This follows from the fact that, although we can never be certain about the conditions of and rationale for an attempt, we know that if we do not intervene the decision is irreversible. Thus, 'direct responsibility over a potentially irreversible decision under conditions of uncertainty, suggests a policy of postponement' (Heyd and Bloch, 1981, p. 201). This policy is vindicated by the fact that most failed suicides are glad that their lives were saved (British Medical Association, 1988). The ethical weight in this area therefore seems to fall heavily on the medical policy which runs counter to putting absolute value on patient autonomy. This means, unfortunately, that we will act inappropriately for the 'Ednas and Arthurs' that fall into our path.

Again we see an intuitive awareness of the realities of human psychology in our policy in this area. People are, in general, not clearcut forward planners who have an autonomously formulated and rationally justified agenda to pursue in their life events. They feel things and react to things in a myriad ways which change over time, and through the vicissitudes of relationships and adverse circumstances. Those patients who are psychologically disturbed are particularly vulnerable to instability in their thoughts and intentions, and therefore require special 'parentalistic' concern. Within the 'shifting sand' of the disturbed psyche, some patterns are relatively stable and others are transient, and thus, in clinical practice, we should try to empower the patient as best we can to look to his abiding interests and to survive the threats to life and well-being posed by his illness.

Reproduction, sexuality, and mental impairment

Leah is a mentally retarded young woman of twenty-five who has a mental age of a five-year-old. She has irregular heavy periods and gets ill when she is given Depo contraception. She enjoys playing with dolls and babies, and is sexually aware to the extent that she has been observed petting with a young male patient that she knows, and has made obviously sexual approaches to other men. Her parents find her periods hard to cope with and do not see hormonal treatment as an answer to her needs. They have asked that she be sterilized by tubal ligation.

The ethical issues in this area are clouded by claims about the human right to reproduce and discrimination against the disabled. To resolve these issues, we need to keep firmly in mind the fact that clinical decisions ought to be made in the best interests of the patient, or with regard to what would be of substantial benefit to the patient, when the patient herself is not competent to make decisions. Here, the patient is clearly not competent and, indeed, is regarded in law as being vulnerable in the area of sexuality. This means that someone else must make these highly value-laden decisions for the patient. Common sense dictates that a patient such as Leah could not care for a baby, nor could she understand or prepare herself for childbirth. She should therefore be protected from this experience as her mental age would suggest. For this reason, and because her mental impairment is a permanent condition, it would seem to be in her best interests to sterilize her, a decision which has been endorsed by courts in Britain and elsewhere (Skegg, 1988). In fact, in most commonwealth jurisdictions, it is thought appropriate to leave the decision to the doctors and the parents of the child as long as they are in agreement. In that there is no reason to suspect that such parents are acting contrary to the best interests of the child, and that it seems reasonable to spare a child the problems of pregnancy and childbirth, this would seem to be the right stand to take.

There are, however, other arguments for the sterilization of the insane or mentally infirm that are not ethically acceptable. The idea that the mentally impaired should be denied any rights to sexual expression or reproduction solely because they are defective and could corrupt the gene pool is one such argument, based as much in discriminatory and stigmatizing beliefs as in any consideration for their real interests and role in society. Similar doubts can be raised about the contention that mentally defective people as a group are generally unfit to be social parents. It would need to be shown that there was real cause to believe that a particular couple were not fit, and would be likely to harm their child or themselves in some way, before the ethical aspects of the decision would be clear. It may well be that in an appropriate setting, a mentally defective couple could provide a standard of parenting that was fair on any offspring they might have, and on others affected by their decision. Thus, we cannot ethically justify the sterilization of the mentally infirm as a general policy. Each case must be considered on the basis of what would be best for the persons concerned. In as much as the affected persons often include parents or other caregivers, they ought to be involved in the decision. The fact that any child produced will also be a member of our society with her own rights means that her interests are also relevant.

Conclusion

We have discussed a number of areas of clinical care in which the psychiatric patient is vulnerable and cannot adequately be covered by the normal ethical considerations governing relations between health care personnel and patients. Special care must be taken to ensure that the patient does not suffer because of the lack of capacity for autonomy and informed decision-making. To this end, there is a presumption in favour of treatment where a treatment offers significant chance of benefit. However, there must also be a constant awareness of the danger of 'locking the patient in' to a stereotype which can lead to disempowering, loss of dignity and chronic dependency beyond what is required for an effective therapeutic relationship. The underlying aim of all psychiatric treatment should be, just as it is in other areas of health care, to restore the patient to full functioning as completely as possible.

Chapter 11

Ethics, etiquette, and malpractice

Introduction

The medical profession is often perceived as closing ranks in the face of any challenge so that the public cannot obtain redress or satisfaction when something goes wrong. Many pathetic case histories point to a tragic lack of regard for the fears and uncertainties of patients and the subsequent unsatisfactory information given in response to a complaint. When a clinical relationship gives rise to this kind of problem, there is often a great deal of publicity focused on the profession and its regulation, but we should remember that such cases represent a tiny proportion of the myriad medical transactions that occur in different settings every day. Despite their relative infrequency, problems of professional discipline pose ethical questions which are being urged more and more forcefully each year by a patient population which is becoming increasingly aware of its own role and importance in the delivery of health care. Should the doctors set the standards? Should they have a code of professional etiquette which sets them apart from other members of society? How should we regulate the profession and deal with bad practice? Should patients have recourse to legal remedy as a means of disciplining doctors and weeding out those who do not practice properly?

The need for standards

We have already noted that those initiated into the knowledge and skills proper to medical practice were set apart, historically, by their readiness to swear an oath that they would put their patients' interests before their own, seek always to try to help and never to harm. It was on this basis that they formed a group who could be trusted to do things to other people which would normally be quite unacceptable. It is implicitly recognized by patients individually, and the public at large, that many of the factors influencing medical decisions are difficult to understand, and require considerable training and experience to master. This implies that there should be a knowledgeable and expert medical body which sets standards for the profession so that the care which any society receives from its practitioners is as good as it can reasonably be expected to be. The mechanism which achieves this goal is the licensing body and the statute law governing professional registration.

In the Commonwealth countries, a person is licensed to practise as a medical practitioner on completing both an approved course of medical education and a period of supervised practice as a doctor. This is normally in a public hospital where one works as part of a team with more senior doctors, and is given responsibilities commensurate with one's knowledge and experience. For specialist recognition, for example as a surgeon, anaesthetist, psychiatrist or cardiologist, further training is required. This is conducted by the Colleges, such as the Royal Australasian College of Surgeons or the Royal Australasian College of Medicine (which trains general physicians, endocrinologists, cardiologists, neurologists, gastroenterologists, and so on). The New Zealand College of General Practitioners has a similar advanced training programme for General Practice but any medical practitioner can practise as a general practitioner without doing that training. In each case, a professional body with the relevant expertise sets standards for good practice and, in conjunction with the licensing body (e.g. the New Zealand Medical Council), enforces these standards. Other health care professions, such as nursing, also have professional registration and licensing procedures. There are also advanced courses for nurses who specialize in various areas of health care.

Any society can take a great deal of comfort in these measures but, we must quickly add, it is obvious that the bodies concerned are largely made up of health care professionals. In a way this is unavoidable, but it can lead to the feeling that professional regulation is 'a closed shop'. There is no doubt that the need for increased patient or 'lay' representation on such bodies is keenly appreciated by the public at large. There is also no doubt that the standards involved are professional, and a decision as to whether they have been breached will often be a matter of professional judgement. So it is important that our statutory regulatory bodies be well balanced and include experienced and informed professional opinion as well as lay representation. Only in this way can we be sure that the decisions made are really in the best interests of the patients who are being protected by them.

Ethics, etiquette, and discipline

Why should there be professional etiquette in medicine? Why should conventions about 'advertising, public statements, setting up in practice . . . and doctor–doctor relationships' have any role in a society where people can make their own choices, and there are already problems with the formation of professional élites? Why, for instance, do we insist on certain protocols governing referral of patients for treatment by different doctors?

> Lorna is fifty and has been attending her doctor, Dr A, for rectal bleeding and indigestion. He has diagnosed piles and irritable bowel syndrome. Eventually Dr A sends her to the outpatients clinic at the public hospital. She is found to have a rectal mass at 20cm from the anal rim and is told that she will be sent an appointment. She is also advised by one of the resident staff to find another GP; he says that he will send his letter to the new GP when she advises the department who that is to be. She rings Dr B to see if she can see him and is told he will take her as a patient. Meanwhile, the hospital notifies her to come into hospital, she has an operation and is discharged home, apparently well, nine days postoperatively. She develops severe abdominal pain on the weekend after her discharge and tries to get a GP to see her. She does not phone Dr A because she thinks he will be annoyed at her for not wanting to come back to him. Dr B has not got her on his practice list and his locum does not go to see her. She presents back at the hospital, extremely unwell, after forty-eight hours of pain which she has attempted to treat with the pain relief she has been given. Lorna is found to have a bowel obstruction, peritonitis and septic shock.

Lorna has suffered from a breakdown of doctor–doctor relationships. The hospital should have acknowledged and replied to the referral from Dr A, and had no business to collude in an irregular transfer of the patient between primary care teams. But Lorna also shows us that the way doctors can take a proprietal and paternal interest in patients (so that they feel reticent about discussing their difficulties) can hinder orderly clinical practice. The orderly conduct of affairs between doctors is supposed to avoid this kind of damaging mix-up in the treatment of patients.

Other provisions are justified on similar grounds and should always be relativized to the best interests of the patients concerned. Actions which can cause problems in the orderly delivery of patient care include deprecating other doctors, advertising, or canvassing patients. The first of these can lead to a breakdown of co-operative care relationships and respectful consultation between doctors with differing expertise. This leads to unsatisfactory patterns of referral, so that patients do not always get health care supported by the best advice that is available. When a profession is seen to allow petty squabbles and inter-professional tensions of the type that deprecating colleagues can lead to, then not only can patterns of care go wrong, but patients themselves can be subjected to groundless anxieties and misapprehensions about those who are treating them. The other types of breach of etiquette give rise to problems because of the lack of checks and balances on the information and professional care arrangements that result.

> Mike has headaches. He reads in his local paper that a new doctor in his area, Dr D, has specialized in the study of headaches and stress syndromes and he decides to see him rather than his own GP, Dr C. Dr D diagnoses Mike as suffering from stress and begins to treat him. Mike's wife is not so sure but, even though the headache is getting worse, Mike reassures her that Dr D is a real expert and knows more than the doctors who do not specialize. Therefore, there is no need to seek further advice. Mike collapses in front of the TV one night and is admitted to hospital for the series of epileptic fits which follow. He dies during one of the subsequent seizures and is found to have a parietal meningioma which has caused fitting and tentorial herniation of the temporal lobe due to raised CO_2 during the seizure.

Advertising allows false claims of expertise to run unchecked by the normal insistence on professional standards of knowledge and skill that have characterized health care in the past. The media are not subject to scientific or professional review and can print what they like about medical practices or supposed treatments. Only where there is careful professional scrutiny, proper licensing provisions, and orderly patterns of practice can patients be sure that they will receive considered information about the availability of care.

The system of relationships which we call professional etiquette is supposed to safeguard these aspects of health care so that patients are not disadvantaged. Unfortunately, on occasion, the professional cohesion of organized medicine has operated to protect from accountability to the public those within the profession who act in ways that are incompatible with this overall ethical requirement.

Incompetence, negligence, incapacity, and misconduct

Doctors can make mistakes for a number of reasons. Some mistakes in treating patients occur because the doctor does not know what he is doing, or cannot do it properly. These are both forms of incompetence, and they result in the doctor not conducting himself properly in his professional capacity. Other problems arise when the doctor does not take due care in some decision or treatment, and consequently delivers a substandard level of professional service. This amounts to negligence. A moral philosopher would be likely to regard the latter sin greater than the former because incompetence seems to be more a lack of skill than a moral failing. But it is clear that in medicine we must consider first and foremost what impact a given defect in care has on the patient, and it is also clear that practising in an incompetent and dangerous manner is just as reprehensible as practising carelessly.

Quite a different kind of problem arises when a doctor is incapacitated to the point that he cannot act properly in his professional duties. This happens as a result of ill-health, which may be psychiatric or physical. In either case, the profession undertakes a duty not only to care for the doctor but also to safeguard his patients. In most developed countries, there is some system in place to detect and treat the sick or impaired doctor so as to ensure that patients are not harmed. This usually involves efforts to help, and provide needed treatment and relief from clinical duties, without the invocation of any professional sanctions in the first instance. It is usually only when the doctor concerned will not take advice that the licensing body can act to restrict or suspend his practice until they are satisfied that he is fit to undertake the professional duties proper to his role.

The last point introduces an important concept in the analysis of professional misconduct. A doctor or health care professional is expected to undertake care only to the extent that he or she is competent to do so. Thus, unethical behaviour can arise, not because the doctor is guilty of malintent, but just because he or she is injudicious.

Mrs T is a competent general surgeon. She is asked to see a young man who has suffered a head injury and been admitted to the local hospital. He is six hours from his injury and has not really roused to the extent expected. She orders a CAT scan which shows an acute subdural haematoma pressing on the brain. She diagnoses the blood clot but fails to distinguish between a subdural and an extradural haematoma. She reassesses the patient and notes that he has not really deteriorated, and so decides to ring the local neurosurgeon. In fact, she would rather do the operation herself as she has always enjoyed the operations she has done for intracranial haematomas, even though she is not really experienced. She makes the phone call and explains the situation stating that she was intending to do the operation herself. The neurosurgeon offers to take over the patient, but finally concurs with Mrs T.

Mrs T attempts the operation but realizes that she is dealing with a subdural haematoma and panics a little. She opens the dura over a limited area and finds that the brain keeps bulging out at her and that she cannot remove the blood clot at all effectively. She resects a certain amount of brain tissue which causes further bleeding before eventually closing up. The patient spends quite a long time in the intensive care unit but eventually survives with partial loss of the use of his right arm and a profound deficit of speech function. The family initiate an inquiry into his care which culminates in disciplinary proceedings.

The council find both Mrs T and the neurosurgeon guilty of professional misconduct. She is guilty because she acted in a way that exceeded her competence, when a reasonable doctor in her position would have taken the alternative of referral to the competent specialist who was available. The neurosurgeon was found wanting in that he implicitly delegated a procedure to someone who did not have the necessary training or experience. His fault was judged substantially less as he had offered to take over the care of the patient, and there was some uncertainty about whether he could reasonably have been expected to know about Mrs T's competence.

This case illustrates the carefully charted and somewhat informally understood lines of responsibility for the delivery of care adequate to meet the needs of a patient. It is because there is a protocol or etiquette to the conduct and transfer of professional duties that we can be clear where our ethical responsibilities lie. The other point that emerges for some from cases of this sort is the propriety of dealing with ethical problems by a mechanism run by the professional organization whose members are under scrutiny.

Two systems of redress

Tort and medical damages are dealt with by one of two different kinds of system in developed countries. First, there are disciplinary systems of the kind which operate in New Zealand, which carry the burden for detecting and dealing with bad medical practice. This can be supplemented with, or effectively supplanted by, a tort-based system in which patients sue their doctors if they believe the doctor has been at fault in delivering poor care which has resulted in their suffering. If such a civil litigation system is the dominant means of redress for medical damages, then the awards made by courts as a result of such suits are the way in which compensation is given to patients who suffer. The alternative is to compensate patients for their injuries and settle the faults relating to matters of professional misconduct by other means. There is no evidence that either system produces, in general, better medical care or less injustice with respect to patients' complaints. There are, however, some cogent reasons to prefer one over the other.

First, the tort system does not differentially punish bad doctors but rather causes any doctor, whether she is at fault or not, a great deal of trouble, anxiety, and inconvenience. It does not punish the bad doctors because the penalties imposed — damages settlements — are paid for by medical malpractice insurance and therefore spread over all contributing doctors. These ultimately result in increased costs to all patients. There is no doubt that the case itself is a major punishment, but that happens to the doctor whether or not she is proven to be at fault. Thus, the system does not serve as an effective means of redress against bad practice.

Second, the doctors found at fault are those who cannot defend their treatment as being as good as would be expected. This is, of course, a matter of expert opinion, and a lay court has no way of distinguishing real experts in a given field from highly qualified but inexpert witnesses. Thus, the lay court is influenced by many facts extraneous to the actual medical realities of the situation and their decision cannot be relied upon to take informed note of those realities.

Third, the kinds of doctors most vulnerable are those who are inexperienced or pioneering. In either case, it is not clear that we wish to punish those who have done their best in an inherently uncertain situation where it will be impossible for them to deny that somebody else who was more experienced or less enterprising might have avoided the bad outcome. We need surgical training, and we need new techniques to be pioneered, but a tort-based system puts definite barriers in the way of both of these aims.

Fourth, the sums of money involved in litigation and damages are immense, and have an appreciable direct and indirect effect on the health bill. Their direct effect is by increasing practice costs for certain specialities to the point where patients must pay large fees to cover them. Their indirect effect is by encouraging doctors to avoid blame by doing everything possible. Having done a test and found it negative, one is more secure before an ill-informed lay court, than if one has to plead careful medical judgement in deciding that a test was not indicated. The impression created by having a 'ticked off' list of detailed (and expensive) investigations is much more positive to the untutored medical ear than the impression created when a clinician justifies not doing one test after another (even if they all ultimately proved irrelevant) on the basis of his own judgement.

Fifth, under a system which awards damages based on successful suits, the patient receives no compensation for injury, no matter how debilitated, unless he proves that his doctor was at fault. This means that two people with identical burdens to bear may have vastly different outcomes from compensation for their injuries, depending on the not-always-well-informed opinion of a group of unqualified judges. This is patently unjust.

For all these reasons, it is probably best to separate the means of compensation for injury from the adjudication of disciplinary matters and professional standards of practice. The medical profession commands the expertise to deliver sound judgements on the clinical conduct of its members, so it should be left to do so. The burden of compensation for injury is ultimately going to be borne by the patient population, whichever way claims are settled, so it is best to make sure that what we all pay for is distributed in a just way and not as a result of a legal lottery in which inexpert people are asked to make difficult decisions about events, the review of which requires considerable expert knowledge and experience.

Regulation and monopolies

A continuing problem for the regulation of the profession is the opposition which arises when medicine becomes a big money-earning enterprise. The restriction of practice to accord with professional standards can then be considered a kind of restriction of trade, and suits can be brought against the licensing bodies on the basis that they are exercising an unfair monopoly. It should be clear from what we have already outlined that this is a gross parody of the real situation and can be given no ethical support whatever. A monopoly exists when one party excludes another party from offering goods and services which would compete for the market. However, in medicine, the services provided have to be of a very high quality because the overall concern of any health care profession ought to be to do the best for the patient, and not to compete in a market. Thus, there must be some check within the system apart from purely competitive forces with all the compromises between cost and quality that they introduce. We must insist upon a powerful and active disciplinary mechanism to safeguard patients from unscrupulous and inexpert practices which they themselves may not be able to evaluate.

It is, therefore, completely inappropriate for any licensing or disciplinary process to be linked to the idea of trade or monopoly. A profession in which the knowledge and skills commanded are complex and inaccessible to most of those who need them, where professional judgement is involved in an assessment of the patient's true needs as distinct from her fears, hopes, misapprehensions and uncertainties, and for which there will also be a range of outcomes determined partly by the unique problem that any patient brings, and partly by the expertise of the professional, cannot open itself to deregulation and must always insist upon a system of regulation so as to protect those who are suffering.

It would be inconsistent with the basic ethos of medicine to do otherwise than scrutinize and regulate standards of practice, and do so by recourse to sound and experienced opinion from those whose standards of practice are widely recognized and respected.

Epilogue: ACC and the right to sue

In New Zealand, since 1974, personal damages resulting from medical misadventure have been subject to compensation by the Accident Compensation Corporation (ACC), and the injured party has not been able to sue for damages. Professionals who contribute to the injury of their patients by mismanagement are often seen to be buffered from the consequences of their actions by this removal of the right to sue. This is, however, an illusion. The tort-based system and the damages settlements that result do not provide focused redress against the wrongdoer because the costs are borne by his professional practice insurance, and then passed on in increased medical costs to the patient population in general. Thus, the only effective, directed redress against faulty health care is via a regulatory and disciplinary mechanism regardless of how the patient is compensated.

The ACC does, however, embed a number of areas of unclarity and inequity. To qualify as accidental, an injury arising from medical care must be 'unexpected and undesigned' (ACC Report, 1981). But it is not clear how unexpected a complication must be in order to count as misadventure. A failure to produce a satisfactory outcome, a side-effect knowingly incurred, or a well-known and common complication would seem not to qualify. But, again, one can ask how well-known or common counts as not 'unexpected'. One is faced with the ludicrous possibility that a complication known well enough to be included in the giving of information prior to consent would, on that basis alone, be excluded. It seems from the legal decision given by Mr Justice Bisson that consequences where the risk is slight, the injury grave, the adverse event unforeseen, or the mishap avoidable will all count as falling under the Act (Vennell, 1986). In any event, it would seem that there is a discretionary aspect to the judgment which, properly interpreted in accordance with precedent, will provide just recompense where appropriate.

Quite apart from the fact that the ACC does not remove any real disincentives, it is not true that doctors are protected from legal proceedings by the ACC. A doctor can still be found guilty of a crime where he acts in a manner which endangers his patient's life and/or well-being as a result of serious medical negligence. Section 155 of the Crimes Act states that those who undertake to provide medical or surgical treatment must use 'reasonable knowledge skill and care' (Cole, 1987). Therefore, if it could be shown that a doctor has acted with 'disregard for the life and safety of his patient' (Cole, 1987), this would seem to be grounds, not only for a judgement that the doctor was criminally negligent, but also for the award of punitive damages (damages awarded to a victim to punish the perpetrator of a crime).

References

ACC 'Notes on personal injury by accident 1981' *Accident Compensation Report* pp 242-3.

Almond, B. 1990 'Personal issues and personal dilemmas' in *AIDS A Moral Issue*, Almond, B. (ed.), MacMillan, London, p 166.

Anscombe, E. 1981 'Modern moral philosophy' in *Ethics, Religion and Politics* Blackwells, Oxford, p 28.

Bancroft, J. 1981 'Ethical aspects of sexuality and sex therapy' in *Psychiatric Ethics* Bloch, S. and P. Chodoff (eds), Oxford University Press, Oxford, p 162.

Barraclough, B., L. Bunch, B. Nelson and P. Sainsbury 1974 'A hundred cases of suicide: clinical aspects' in *British Journal of Psychiatry* 125, pp 355-73.

Beauchamp, T.L., and L. Walters 1989 *Contemporary Issues in Bioethics* 3rd edn., Wadsworth Publishing Company, Belmont, California.

Beecher, H.K. 1970 *Research and the Individual* Little Brown, Boston.

Bok, S. 1980 *Lying: Moral Choice in Public and Private Life* Quartet, London.

British Medical Association 1988 *Euthanasia* BMA, London.

California Supreme Court 1976 'Tarasoff v Regents of the University of California' *Cal Rpt* 14, 551 P 2d 347.

Campbell, A.V. 1984 *Moderated Love: A Theology of Professional Care* SPCK, London.

Campbell, A.V. 1987 'The hospital ethics committee' Guest editorial in *Hospital Therapeutics*, August, pp 5-7.

Cole, D. 1987 *Medical practice and professional conduct in New Zealand* Roydhouse, Carterton, New Zealand.

Coxon, A. 1990 'Coping with the threat of death' in *AIDS A Moral Issue* Almond, B. (ed.), MacMillan, London.

Dansey, H. 1975 'A view of death' in *Te Ao Hurihuri: the world moves on: aspects of Maoritanga* King, M. (ed), Hicks Smith, Wellington, New Zealand.

Deuchar, N. 1984 'AIDS in New York City' *British J. Psychiatry* 145, pp 612-19.

Feinberg, J. 1985 'The mistreatment of dead bodies' *Hastings Center Report* 15 (2), pp 31-7.

Frame, J. 1982 *Faces in the Water* Braziller, USA.

Gaylin, W. 1974 'Harvesting the dead' *Harper's Magazine*, September, pp 23-30.

General Medical Council of Britain 1988 'Advice on testing for HIV infection', *Lancet*, August 20, p 465.

Gillam, L. 1989 'Fetal tissue transplantation: a philosophical approach' in *Proceedings of the Conference: The Fetus as Tissue Donor: Use or Abuse?* Gillam, L., (ed.), Monash University Centre for Human Bioethics, Melbourne pp 60-66.

Gillett G. 1986 'Why let people die?' *J. Med. Ethics* 12 (2), pp 83-6.

Gillett G. 1987 Reply to J.M. Stanley: 'Fiddling and Clarity' *J. Med Ethics* 13, pp 23-5.

Gillett, G. 1988 'AIDS and confidentiality' *J. of Applied Philosophy* 4 (1), pp 15-20; reprinted in Almond, B. (1990).

Gillett, G. 1989 'HIV and the epidemiologist' *Lancet* November 19, p 1228.

Gillett, G. 1990 'Consciousness, the brain and what matters' *Bioethics* 4, pp 181-98.

Glover, J. 1977 *Causing death and saving lives* Penguin, Harmondsworth.

Hampton, J.R. 1983 *British Medical Journal* 287, p 1237.

Hare, R. 1981 'The philosophical basis of psychiatric ethics' in *Psychiatric Ethics* Bloch, S. and P. Chodoff (eds), Oxford University Press, Oxford, p 44.

Heyd and Bloch 1981 'The ethics of suicide' in *Psychiatric Ethics*, Bloch, S. and P. Chodoff (eds), Oxford University Press, Oxford.

Higgs, R. 1985 'On telling patients the truth' in *Moral Dilemmas in Modern Medicine* Lockwood, M. (ed), Oxford University Press, Oxford pp 187-202.

Iglesias, T. 1984 'In vitro fertilisation; the major issues' *Journal of Medical Ethics* 10, pp 32-7.

Illich, I. 1977 *Limits to Medicine* Penguin, London.

Jones, D.G. 1987 *Manufacturing Humans* Inter-Varsity Press, Leicester.

Jones, D.G. 1989 'Brain birth and personal identity' *Journal of Medical Ethics* 15, pp 173-8.

Jones, D.G. 1989 *Brain Grafts* Grove Books, Bramcote, Nottingham.

Jones, D.G. 1991 'Fetal neural transplantation: placing the ethical debate within the context of society's use of human material' *Bioethics* 5, pp 23-43.

Jones, D.G. and S. Fennell 1991 'Bequests, cadavers and dissections: sketches from New Zealand history' *New Zealand Medical Journal* 104, pp 210-12.

Jones, D.G. and B. Telfer 1990 'National bioethics committees: developments and prospects' *New Zealand Medical Journal* 103, pp 66-8.

Kant, I. 1785 *Fundamental Principles of the Metaphysic of Morals* N.Y. Liberal Arts Press, 1949.

Kant, I. 1963 *Lectures on ethics* (trsl. L. Infield) Harper & Row, New York.

Karasu, T. 1981 'Ethical aspects of psychotherapy' in *Psychiatric Ethics* Bloch, S. and P. Chodoff (eds), Oxford University Press, Oxford.

Kesey, K. 1962 *One Flew Over The Cuckoo's Nest* Viking Penguin, USA.

Kirby, J.M., 1989 'Legal implications of AIDS' in *Legal implications of AIDS*, Paterson, R. (ed), Legal Research Foundation, Auckland.

Kleinig. J. 1985 *Ethical Issues in Psychosurgery* George Allen & Unwin, London.

Kubler-Ross, E. 1969 *On Death and Dying* Macmillan, New York.

Laing, R.D. 1965 *The Divided Self* Penguin, Harmondsworth.

Lancet editorial, 17 November 1832, pp 243-5.

Langerak, E.A. 1979 'Abortion: listening to the middle' *Hastings Center Report 9* (5), pp 24-8.

Leenen, H.J.J. 1987 'Euthanasia, assistance to suicide and the law: developments in the Netherlands' *Health Policy* 8, pp 197-206.

Marcus R. and The CDC Cooperative Needlestick Surveillance Group 1988 'Surveillance of health care workers exposed to blood from patients with the human immunodeficiency virus' *New Eng. J. Med.* 319, pp 1118-23.

Max, D. 1989 'This and that: the ethics of experimentation' *Trends in Pharmacological Sciences* 10, pp 133-5.

Maxwell, R. 1974 *Health Care: The Growing Dilemma* McKinsey & Co., New York.

May, W.F. 1983 *Physician's Covenant: Images of the Healer in Medical Ethics* Westminster Press, Philadelphia.

May, W.F. 1985 'Religious justification for donating body parts' *Hastings Center Report* 15 (2)/5. pp 38-42.

McCormick, R.A. 1981 *How Brave a New World?* Doubleday, New York.

McGarry, L. and P. Chodoff 1981 'The ethics of involuntary hospitalisation' in *Psychiatric Ethics* Bloch, S. and P. Chodoff (eds), Oxford University Press, Oxford, p 217.

Medical Council of New Zealand June 1990 *A Statement for the Medical Profession on Information and Consent.*

Moe, K. 1984 'Should the Nazi research data be cited?' *Hastings Center Report* 14 (6), pp 5-7.

Murphy, G. E. 1973 'Suicide and the right to die' *Am. J. Psychiatry* 130, pp 472-3.

New Zealand Health Department 1991 *National Standard for Area Health Board Ethics Committees.*

Newkirk, I. 1986 'Who will live, who will die?' quoted in K. McCabe *Washingtonian Magazine*, August, p. 115.

Pappworth, M.H. 1967 *Human Guinea Pigs: Experimentation on Man* Routledge & Kegan Paul, London.

Pellegrino, E.D. and D.S. Thomasma 1981 *A Philosophical Basis of Medical Practice* Oxford University Press, Oxford.

Pellegrino, E.D. and D.S. Thomasma 1988 *For the Patient's Good* Oxford University Press, Oxford.

Pinching, A. 1990 'AIDS: clinical and scientific background' in *AIDS a Moral Issue* Almond, B. (ed), MacMillan, London.

Poplawski, N. and G. Gillett 1991 'Ethics and embryos' *Journal of Medical Ethics* 17, pp 62-9.

President's Commission 1983 *Deciding to forego life-sustaining treatment* U.S. Govt Printing Office, pp 174-5.

Rachels, J. 1975 'Active and passive euthanasia' *New England J. Med.* 292, pp 78-80.

Rawls, J. 1971 *A Theory of Justice* Oxford University Press, Oxford.

Reich, W. 1981 'Psychiatric diagnosis as an ethical problem' in *Psychiatric Ethics* Bloch, S. and P. Chodoff (eds), Oxford University Press, Oxford.

Report of the Committee of Inquiry into Human Fertilisation and Embryology (Warnock Committee) 1984, London, Her Majesty's Stationery Office:

Peel Committee Report (1972) in Britain

National Commission for the Protection of Human Subjects of Biomedical and Behavioural Research (1975) in USA

National Health and Medical Research Council (1984) in Australia

Review of the Guidance on the Research Use of Fetuses and Fetal Material (Polkinghorne Committee) 1989, London, Her Majesty's Stationery Office.

Richardson, R. 1988 *Death, Dissection and the Destitute* Penguin Books, London.

Rollin, B.E. 1989 *The Unheeded Cry* Oxford University Press, Oxford.

Royal Society 1990 *The Case for Human Embryological Research* Royal Society, London.

Seneca 1920 *Epistua Morales* (Vol II) (trsl. R.M. Grumere) Harvard University Press, Cambridge, Massachusetts.

Singer, P. 1975 *Animal Liberation* New York Review/Random House, New York.

Singer, P. 1983 'Sanctity of life or quality of life?' *Paediatrics* 72 (1), July, pp 274-8.

Singer, P. and D. Wells 1984 *The Reproduction Revolution* Oxford University Press, Oxford.

Skegg, D.C.G. 1989 'Heterosexually acquired HIV infection' *British Medical Journal* 298, pp 401-2.

Skegg, P.D.G. 1988 *Law, Ethics and Medicine* Clarendon Press, Oxford.

Smithurst, M. 1990 'AIDS: risk and discrimination' in *AIDS a Moral Issue*, Almond, B. (ed), McMillan, London, p 103.

Sommers, C.H. 1985 'Tooley's immodest proposal' *The Hastings Center Report* 15 (3), pp 39-42.

Storr, A. 1970 *Human Aggression* Penguin Books, London.

Szasz, T. 1983 'Objections to psychiatry' in *States of mind* Miller, J. (ed.) BBC, London.

Tolstoy, L. 1960 *The Death of Ivan Ilyich* Penguin Books, London p. 126.

Tooley, M. 1983 *Abortion and Infanticide* Clarendon Press, Oxford.

Veatch, R.M. 1981 *A Theory of Medical Ethics* Part II, Basic Books, New York.

Vennell, M. 1986 *Recent Law* 12, pp 42-3.

Walters, L. 1979 'Human in vitro fertilization: a review of the ethical literature' *Hastings Center Report* 9 (4), pp 23-43.

Wennberg, R. 1985 *Life in the Balance* Eerdmans, Grand Rapids.

Williams, B. 1985 *Ethics and the Limits of Philosophy* Collins, London, p 1.

Wolsterstorff, N. 1978 *Lament for a Son* Eerdmans, Grand Rapids.

Appendix I

Codes of Ethics

The Hippocratic Oath

I swear by Apollo the healer, invoking all the gods and goddesses to be my witnesses, that I will fulfil this Oath and this written Covenant to the best of my ability and judgement.

I will look upon him who shall have taught me this Art even as one of my parents. I will share my substance with him, and I will supply his necessities, if he be in need. I will regard his offspring even as my own brethren, and I will teach them this Art, if they would learn it, without fee or covenant. I will impart this Art by precept, by lecture and by every mode of teaching, not only to my own sons but to the sons of him who taught me, and to disciples bound by covenant and oath, according to the Law of Medicine.

The regimen I adopt shall be for the benefit of the patients according to my ability and judgement, and not for their hurt or for any wrong. I will give no deadly drug to any, though it be asked of me, nor will I counsel such, and especially I will not aid a woman to procure abortion. Whatsoever house I enter, there will I go for the benefit of the sick, refraining from all wrongdoing or corruption, and especially from any act of seduction, of male or female, of bond or free. Whatsoever things I see or hear concerning the life of men, in my attendance on the sick or even apart therefrom, which ought not to be noised abroad, I will keep silence thereon, counting such things to be as sacred secrets. Pure and holy will I keep my Life and my Art.

If I fulfil this Oath and confound it not, be it mine to enjoy Life and Art alike, with good repute among all men at all times. If I transgress and violate my oath, may the reverse be my lot.

The Geneva Convention Code of Medical Ethics

Adopted by the World Medical Association in 1949
I solemnly pledge myself to consecrate my life to the service of humanity;
I will give to my teachers the respect and gratitude which is their due;
I will practice my profession with conscience and dignity;
The health of my patient will be my first consideration;

I will respect the secrets which are confided in me;
I will maintain by all the means in my power, the honour and the noble traditions of the medical profession;
My colleagues will be my brothers;
I will not permit considerations of religion, nationality, race, party politics or social standing to intervene between my duty and my patient.
I will maintain the utmost respect for human life from the time of conception; even under threat. I will not use my medical knowledge contrary to the laws of humanity.
I make these promises solemnly, freely and upon my honour.

Council for International Organizations of Medical Sciences (CIOMS)

International Guiding Principles for Biomedical Research Involving Animals, June 1984

1 Basic Principles

I. The advancement of biological knowledge and the development of improved means for the protection of the health and well-being both of man and of animals require recourse to experimentation on intact live animals of a wide variety of species.

II. Methods such as mathematical models, computer simulation and *in vitro* biological systems should be used wherever appropriate.

III. Animal experiments should be undertaken only after due consideration of their relevance for human or animal health and the advancement of biological knowledge.

IV. The animals selected for an experiment should be of an appropriate species and quality, and the minimum number required, to obtain scientifically valid results.

V. Investigators and other personnel should never fail to treat animals as sentient, and should regard their proper care and use and the avoidance or minimization of discomfort, distress, or pain as ethical imperatives.

VI. Investigators should assume that procedures that would cause pain in human beings cause pain in other vertebrate species although more needs to be known about the perception of pain in animals.

VII. Procedures with animals that may cause more than momentary or minimal pain or distress should be performed with appropriate sedation, analgesia, or anesthesia in accordance with accepted veterinary practice. Surgical or other painful procedures should not be performed on unanesthetized animals paralysed by chemical agents.

VIII. Where waivers are required in relation to the provisions of article VII, the decisions should not rest solely with the investigators directly concerned but should be made, with due regard to the provisions of articles IV, V, and VI, by a suitably constituted review body. Such waivers should not be made solely for the purposes of teaching or demonstration.

IX. At the end of, or, when appropriate, during an experiment, animals that would otherwise suffer severe or chronic pain, distress, discomfort, or disablement that cannot be relieved should be painlessly killed.

X. The best possible living conditions should be maintained for animals kept for biomedical purposes. Normally the care of animals should be under the supervision of veterinarians having experience in laboratory animal science. In any case, veterinary care should be available as required.

XI. It is the responsibility of the director of an institute or department using animals to ensure that investigators and personnel have appropriate qualifications or experience for conducting procedures on animals. Adequate opportunities shall be provided for in-service training, including the proper and humane concern for the animals under their care.

World Medical Association Declaration of Helsinki

Recommendations guiding physicians in biomedical research involving human subjects
Adopted by the 18th World Medical Assembly, Helsinki, Finland, June 1964 and amended by the 29th World Medical Assembly, Tokyo, Japan, October 1975, 35th World Medical Assembly, Venice, Italy, October 1983, and the 41st World Medical Assembly, Hong Kong, September 1989.

Introduction:

It is the mission of the physician to safeguard the health of the people. His or her knowledge and conscience are dedicated to the fulfilment of this mission.

The Declaration of Geneva of the World Medical Association binds the physician with the words, 'The health of my patient will be my first consideration', and the International Code of Medical Ethics declares that, 'A physician shall act only in the patient's interest when providing medical care which might have the effect of weakening the physical and mental condition of the patient'.

The purpose of biomedical research involving human subjects must be to improve diagnostic, therapeutic and prophylactic procedures and the understanding of the aetiology and pathogenesis of disease.

In current medical practice most diagnostic, therapeutic or prophylactic procedures involve hazards. This applies especially to biomedical research.

Medical progress is based on research which ultimately must rest in part on experimentation involving human subjects.

In the field of biomedical research a fundamental distinction must be recognized between medical research in which the aim is essentially diagnostic or therapeutic for a patient, and medical research, the essential object of which is purely scientific and without implying direct diagnostic or therapeutic value to the person subjected to the research.

Special caution must be exercised in the conduct of research which may affect the environment, and the welfare of animals used for research must be respected.

Because it is essential that the results of laboratory experiments be applied to human beings to further scientific knowledge and to help suffering humanity, the World Medical Association has prepared the following recommendations as a guide to every physician in biomedical research involving human subjects. They should be kept under review in the future. It must be stressed that the standards as drafted are only a guide to physicians all over the world. Physicians are not relieved from criminal, civil and ethical responsibilities under the laws of their own countries.

I   Basic Principles

1.   Biomedical research involving human subjects must conform to generally accepted scientific principles and should be based on adequately performed laboratory and animal experimentation and on a thorough knowledge of the scientific literature.

2.   The design and performance of each experimental procedure involving human subjects should be clearly formulated in an experimental protocol which should be transmitted for consideration, comment and guidance to a specially appointed committee independent of the investigator and the sponsor provided that this independent committee is in conformity with the laws and regulations of the country in which the research experiment is performed.

3.   Biomedical research involving human subjects should be conducted only by scientifically qualified persons and under the supervision of a clinically competent medical person. The responsibility for the human subject must always rest with a medically qualified person and never rest on the subject of the research, even though the subject has given his or her consent.

4.   Biomedical research involving human subjects cannot legitimately be carried out unless the importance of the objective is in proportion to the inherent risk to the subject.

5.   Every biomedical research project involving human subjects should be preceded by careful assessment of predictable risks in comparison with foreseeable benefits to the subject or to others. Concern for the interests of the subject must always prevail over the interests of science and society.

6.   The right of the research subject to safeguard his or her integrity must always be respected. Every precaution should be taken to respect the privacy of the subject and to minimize the impact of the study on the subject's physical and mental integrity and on the personality of the subject.

7.   Physicians should abstain from engaging in research projects involving human subjects unless they are satisfied that the hazards involved are believed to be predictable. Physicians should cease any investigation if the hazards are found to outweigh the potential benefits.

8.   In publication of the results of his or her research, the physician is obliged to preserve the accuracy of the results. Reports of experimentation not in accordance with the principles laid down in this Declaration should not be accepted for publication.

9. In any research on human beings, each potential subject must be adequately informed of the aims, methods, anticipated benefits and potential hazards of the study and the discomfort it may entail. He or she should be informed that he or she is at liberty to abstain from participation in the study and that he or she is free to withdraw his or her consent to participation at any time. The physician should then obtain the subject's freely-given informed consent, preferably in writing.

10. When obtaining informed consent for the research project the physician should be particularly cautious if the subject is in a dependent relationship to him or her or may consent under duress. In that case the informed consent should be obtained by a physician who is not engaged in the investigation and who is completely independent of this official relationship.

11. In case of legal incompetence, informed consent should be obtained from the legal guardian in accordance with national legislation. Where physical or mental incapacity makes it impossible to obtain informed consent, or when the subject is a minor, permission from the responsible relative replaces that of the subject in accordance with national legislation.

    Whenever the minor child is in fact able to give a consent, the minor's consent must be obtained in addition to the consent of the minor's legal guardian.

12. The research protocol should always contain a statement of the ethical considerations involved and should indicate that the principles enunciated in the present Declaration are complied with.

II Medical Research Combined with Professional Case (Clinical Research)

1. In the treatment of the sick person, the physician must be free to use a new diagnostic and therapeutic measure, if in his or her judgement it offers hope of saving life, re-establishing health or alleviating suffering.

2. The potential benefits, hazards and discomfort of a new method should be weighed against the advantages of the best current diagnostic and therapeutic methods.

3. In any medical study, every patient – including those of a control group, if any – should be assured of the best proven diagnostic and therapeutic method.

4. The refusal of the patient to participate in a study must never interfere with the physician—patient relationship.

5. If the physician considers it essential not to obtain informed consent, the specific reasons for this proposal should be stated in the experimental protocol for transmission to the independent committee (1, 2).

6. The physician can combine medical research with professional care, the objective being the acquisition of new medical knowledge, only to the extent that medical research is justified by its potential diagnostic or therapeutic value for the patient.

III Non-therapeutic Biomedical Research Involving Human Subjects (Non-clinical Biomedical Research)

1. In the purely scientific application of medical research carried out on a human being, it is the duty of the physician to remain the protector of the life and health of that person on whom biomedical research is being carried out.

2. The subjects should be volunteers – either healthy persons or patients for whom the experimental design is not related to the patient's illness.

3. The investigator or the investigating team should discontinue the research if in his/her or their judgement it may, if continued, be harmful to the individual.

4. In research on man, the interest of science and society should never take precedence over considerations related to the well-being of the subject.

Appendix II

Biculturalism and New Zealand medical ethics

New Zealand society is a mixture of two cultures and therefore its health-care system ought to reflect and be accountable to the norms of both. But issues that arise are not peculiar to a New Zealand context because many societies must develop medical ethics in a way that reflects the beliefs and concerns of more than one tradition of thought. Multiculturalism tends to have a haphazard, compromise character whereby different traditions agree to live and let live, but indigenous peoples are not always happy with this state of affairs. The Treaty of Waitangi, concluded between the sovereign Māori people of Aotearoa and the British Crown, in fact promised far more than a polyglot marketplace of traditions falling into some uneasy equilibrium. The Treaty meant that the value and integrity of the Māori people were considered important in the development of a bicultural society. Thus, New Zealand is distinct in that the orderly governance of the country was settled on the basis that the integrity and treasures of the Māori people would be assured. The problems that this historic agreement is facing in policy areas (including health care) therefore, are similar to and yet different from those of other multicultural societies. The point that must be emphasized is that taha Māori (the Māori perspective) should be an integral part of the ethos of New Zealand health care.

For those of us who teach and explore medical ethics, it has been interesting to note the convergence between the concerns of certain strands of philosophical ethics and the concerns of Māori people. Both medical ethics and Māori thought recognize the importance of respect for the individual as not just a patient but also a being with feelings and standing of her own. Both recognize the fact that health care is concerned not solely with physiological interventions. However, there are some distinct emphases which a Māori perspective on health introduces and which should be included in our understanding of clinical ethics. Our suspicion is that many of these distinctive insights are shared by other indigenous peoples.

The Māori perspective on illness regards physical ills as not completely separate from mental or spiritual ills. Thus the Māori patient may feel himself not merely to have suffered a physiological or anatomical injury, but to have been wounded and weakened in his soul or essential being as part of his illness. The balance between life and death and the physical body that stands as their centre is symbolic of the meeting of physical and spiritual that lies at the heart of a Māori conception of life. The option of fully secularized humanism, which frames most discussions in contemporary medical ethics, is therefore not open to a view of health care which aims to respect taha Māori. In sickness and death the inseparability of the physical and the spiritual is made vivid. Death is, in fact, at the same time the ending of a life and the sign of reaffirmation of the identity of the person who has died. This identity reaches far back in time and locates the person in a meaningful context so that death is not futile or meaningless.

> If Maui, the greatest culture hero in Māori mythology, could not defeat death, then ordinary humans must surely accept its inevitability. (Walker, p. 36–7)

Sickness, the forerunner of death, has a very special meaning for Māori patients. It reminds them of the context in which individual lives are conducted. A serious illness raises questions about one's readiness for death and one's attitude to things that matter. Therefore sickness is a state in which meaning and identity and the perspective of taha Māori are especially relevant. In this state, the Māori individual is highly dependent on sources of strength aside from her own mana (the divinely-given power of the individual). A potent source of mana is belonging – or the connections between the life of the individual and the life of the whānau (family). This belonging allows a patient in a weakened state to draw strength, courage, and the ability to face her illness from the fact that 'My relation and I are part of the same tree, we share the same ancestry and claims of that ancestry are very real' (Dansey 1975).

The Māori patient lives also with a sense of wholeness as a human being. This intuition rejects the scientific dissection of bodily function into a complex, with varying contributions from different bodily organs and mental faculties. All a person's functions are linked, and all must be in harmony for the patient to function healthily. Of course, some body parts are recognized to have distinctive or special roles in one's function as a human being and therefore are given special significance. These special meanings tend to be expressed in terms of tapu (sacredness, dedication, or the recognition of spiritual significance). Thus the head is tapu in one way, the sexual organs are tapu in another, and so on. The health-care team can convey some very adverse messages by disregarding these tapu and therefore devaluing the person whose body is no longer being treated with due respect. Given the close connection between body and soul, the treatment of one's body as a mere thing may carry the implication for the patient that his mana or individual dignity is similarly reduced, and that the doctors either do not care or that they have realized there is no hope for him. Therefore, doctors should not treat a Māori person, in his physical being, as a mere collection of functioning parts.

It is not only unacceptable to treat the parts of an individual as totally separate functioning units, it is equally unacceptable to treat whole individuals in that way. The non-Māori is reckoned to have an intact sense of his own agenda and interests and to be individually competent to make sound decisions without reference to the underlying spiritual and inclusive reality which, in Māori terms, shows itself in the harm or illness that has befallen him. The all-embracing nature of the sources and significance of this harm, which at one level manifests itself in physical disease, entails that the sick Māori person is not in a position to be autonomous in the Western liberal sense of that word. The Māori patient may not feel confident that she fully understands what is happening to her. She will attempt to read, from the universal body language of her (usually Pākehā) caregivers, the messages that are hard to evaluate from their words. She, like many Pākehā patients, will be asking 'What does this mean for me?', but unlike for some Pākehā, that decision will be embedded in layers of meaning that can only be unpacked in the context of whānau: 'When doubt of identity creeps in, action is paralysed' (Walker, p. 44). Identity, belonging, standing, and mana are all linked in Māori thought. The dependency of the Māori person does not justify paternalism, but rather implies that we must do those things that will empower a Māori patient to take her proper role in the clinical situation and come to terms with illness and health-care decisions in her own way. These things include recognizing the need for support from the whānau, and other relevant mental and spiritual support, when decisions are discussed. The Pākehā doctor is not necessarily able to meet these dependency needs, and may have to defer to customary ways of discussion and interaction. The problems are illustrated in the following case.

James is a 38-year-old Māori carpenter admitted with severe central chest pain. He is found to have ECG evidence of a myocardial infarction. Over the next few days this is confirmed with enzyme studies, and after considering the history, the doctors decide he ought to have a coronary angiogram. The junior doctor explains everything to James, who appears to agree with what is proposed and has no questions to ask. Later she finds that James refuses to sign the consent form, and she is puzzled. The cardiologist in charge of the case is asked about it and says something derogatory about the intelligence of Māori patients in general, claiming that they never seem to know what they want. He confronts James in an aggressive manner and later the nursing staff find James making moves to leave the ward because he does not like that 'specialist fella' and would rather go home.

It is instructive to listen to some of the perceptions and concerns that James has had on his mind throughout these events.[1]

They say it's something wrong with my heart. That is a pretty tapu kind of thing. They tell me that my heart is weak and bits of it might die off. I wonder what a joker is like when his heart has already started to die. They want to put some tube in it with this X-ray dye stuff and they say it might even make it die a little bit more. I don't know about that. I wonder what the old man would say. He knows about these tapu things. Maybe taking the pictures of my heart will really screw things up with old James's mana here. Anyway, I can't say anything to these doctors, not a working bloke like me but I'm not too sure about it. I'm not going to sign this form anyway, that's much too hard to figure out. I've got to talk to somebody, maybe the old man or Aunt Rangi, they will know what a joker ought to do. I think I will go home and talk to them so that that big fella doesn't get so mad any more. I will come back and see that young sheila doctor when we have all had a talk about it.

James's concerns reflect the points we have already listed. He is concerned about the impact of this disease, not only on his physical body, but on his soul or being-as-a-person. The fact that his heart is affected has deep and uncertain significance about the kinds of harms he is suffering and the meanings of his sickness in terms of his identity and mana. To cope with these concerns requires both assurance and personal strength, and any illness weakens a person both physically and psychologically (and, for a Māori person, it indicates a state of spiritual weakening). The fact that it is his heart which is affected only intensifies the importance for James of doing things properly and considering carefully what is correct. James cannot express these concerns in the, for him, isolated context of a Pākehā controlled hospital setting. In that setting he has no tūrangawaewae (status or standing). He does not know how things are done or where he stands because he is not in a place where he belongs. This forces him to search elsewhere for the critical help and guidance he needs, although he realizes that this final decision might be to choose the care plan that the Pākehā doctors offer.

Having said all this, there remains the fact that some Māori patients want to do it the Pākehā way. This should be clear to all concerned but it should never be taken for granted and the opportunity for the whānau or kaumātua (elders) to be involved should always be offered. The difficult cases are those in which the wishes of a Māori individual differ from those of the most obvious support group. In such a case the patient may not wish others to be involved and the health-care team may be in the unfortunate situation of trying to protect the patient's wishes against those that they would normally try to co-operate with and involve. As things stand in New Zealand law and medical ethics, it is not permissible for health-care workers to breach confidentiality against the express wishes of the patients except in the rare cases we have outlined (child abuse, AIDS, dangerous use of a motor vehicle). It would, however, be wise for the health-care workers concerned to involve somebody who can attempt a reconciliation between individual and whānau; this, ultimately, may in itself be a very healing thing to do.

The final concern that biculturalism raises is that of social justice. Māori people are disadvantaged in the competitive world of contemporary urban life where sharing and caring may often lose out badly to economic considerations. Their social mores are co-operative and communal and, in the Treaty of Waitangi, the Crown has agreed implicitly to honour these and to protect them. Honouring the Treaty of Waitangi means that we cannot opt for a user-pays, wealth-based system of health-care delivery. Māori health issues are not only issues of taha Māori, but issues of a group whose identity and tūrangawaewae has been threatened by a foreign set of values and institutions. In addressing that wrong, we will find ourselves addressing broad issues of health-care delivery that are intrinsic to a caring society where people are valued in and for themselves.

All too often, we in modern clinical life arrogantly believe that we do all that is required when we treat each individual as an economic and self-governing unit. Patients are often scared and uncertain, needing trustworthy help and guidance, and we must respect those needs and aim to empower a patient to cope with them and preserve his individual dignity. Trying to understand the fears and concerns of Māori patients will, we believe, open our eyes to the fact that, at heart, people are not ideal, rational, liberal, economic units, and that medicine and ethics both must apply themselves to beings who are needy and vulnerable. Such beings need care, consideration, and relatedness as much as they need any other benefit we might confer on them. This insight should inform clinical ethics in all the difficult areas of health care, and it introduces a perspective which is valuable for contexts quite removed from that of New Zealand biculturalism.

1 We have put these in words that have been used in discussions with Māori patients; there is no intention to indicate anything about the general language and education of Māori people.

Appendix III

Issues in genetics

The term 'genetic engineering' encapsulates people's fears regarding future abuses of science, since it is seen as having the potential to manipulate human nature. For some, it is 'playing God' in the most objectionable way. However, present-day human genetics is far less monolithic than this term suggests, ranging as it does from genetic screening and the use of DNA probes to preemptive intervention and selective abortion; from genetic counselling to somatic and germ line gene therapy; and from the human genome project (with its efforts to produce the complete nucleotide sequence of the human genome) to cloning and eugenics. This range is made possible only because contemporary molecular genetics allows for the manipulation of the genetic content of human cells. Consequently, it holds out prospects both for dramatically extending the range of current medical therapies and for effecting radical changes to the way in which medicine itself is practised. Hitherto intractable genetic diseases, such as cystic fibrosis and muscular dystrophy, are now being unravelled and the genes involved have been defined, while the nature of cancer as an acquired genetic disease is being clarified.

Genetic screening was revolutionized in the late 1970s by the advent of the recombinant DNA technologies, that in turn have led to the development of DNA probes for detecting large numbers of human genetic variants and genes with known functions. The amount of information stemming from these procedures is enormous, and its use demands serious ethical assessment. Criteria are required for determining who is to be tested, and what those with positive tests are to be told and whether their privacy and confidentiality can be maintained under all circumstances. The testing of people for susceptibility to a disease (for instance, severe arthritis or manic depressive illness) can be used sensitively and constructively, but it may serve to stigmatize individuals because of their genetic constitution. The consequence of genetic testing of the foetus is frequently abortion following a positive finding, although the prospects of treatment of afflicted foetuses are improving. The precision of genetic information is not always as great as some claim, and care needs to be exercised to ensure that it does not lead to genetic determinism.

Somatic cell gene therapy, which was first tested in humans in 1989, involves the correction of gene defects in patients' own cells, the cells in question being somatic cells (that is, ordinary body cells). The strategy involves gene replacement, gene correction or gene augmentation, the genes being introduced via retroviral vectors. The aim of this form of gene therapy is to modify a particular cell population and so rectify a particular disease in a particular patient. As such, it is similar to procedures like organ transplantation, but is far more powerful than any indirect genetic therapies. However, there are technical difficulties associated with the expression and appropriate regulation of new genes in somatic cells, and from its current limitation to disorders stemming from defective function of genes in the specialized cells from which blood cells are derived. For some time it will be confined to attempts at correcting single gene defects, such as are found in thalassemia and phenylketonuria.

Since its aim is the alleviation of disease, and not the improvement of the human species, it fits within conventional goals for health care. Ethical issues of significance include the need to balance any potential benefits and harms, and assess the safety and effectiveness of new techniques. There must be unequivocal evidence from animal studies that the inserted gene will function adequately and have no deleterious effects; there needs to be assurance that the new gene can be accurately placed into the target cells and that it will remain there long enough to be effective, that it will be expressed in the cell at the appropriate level and only in that tissue, and that neither it nor the retroviruses will harm the cell or the patient. It is important to assess the benefits of gene therapy against current alternative therapies (such as bone marrow transplantation), and to ensure that the interests of the patients are paramount. For the foreseeable future, it should be viewed as the treatment of last resort.

It may be objected that somatic cell gene therapy is unethical since it represents the beginning of a slippery slope, its inevitable concomitant being germ line gene therapy and eugenics. Understandable as this objection may be, there is a considerable moral gulf between gene therapy to treat disease and gene manipulation to alter behaviour or morality.

Germ line gene therapy involves inserting the gene into the germ line (sperms, eggs, and embryos), so that when the modified individual reproduces all offspring will have the inserted gene instead of the original defective one. It is attempting to manipulate an early embryo so that the individual it will become is not afflicted with a fatal disease. Animal experiments have shown this form of gene therapy to be associated with high risks, since gene expression may occur in inappropriate tissues. Since the foreign gene is inserted randomly into the host DNA, some facets of normal embryological development may be disrupted with serious adverse consequences. Further, any damage to the DNA caused by this procedure will stay in the germ line and be passed on to subsequent generations. But what if it becomes a safe and effective procedure?

Were this to happen, there are various arguments in favour of germ line gene therapy. Some genetic disorders may only be amenable to treatment in this way (for example, brain cells in hereditary central nervous system disorders, which are not open to genetic repair after birth). It would also dispense with the need to repeat somatic cell therapy in different generations of a family with a genetic disorder, by eliminating the defective gene from the population and so improving the efficiency of gene therapy. In assessing these arguments, it is pertinent to point out that germ line therapy involves obtaining embryos via *in vitro* fertilization, determining which ones require treatment, and then carrying out the therapy. However, the far simpler procedure of refraining from implanting defective embryos achieves the same therapeutic aims without running the risks of inserting a new gene into a defective embryo. It is, therefore, far less problematic ethically. This simpler course of action requires the disposal of defective embryos, and may be rejected by some on the grounds that it is unethical to select healthy embryos and reject defective ones. Neither would it satisfy those wishing to eliminate a defective gene from the population.

Enhancement genetic engineering involves the insertion of a gene in an attempt to alter a particular trait of an individual. This approach has ethical problems, since it aims to alter a healthy individual in a permanent manner. This is similar to providing growth hormone to normal individuals in order to improve their sporting prowess. The extra gene (whether normal or modified) may have adverse consequences resulting from protein imbalance. However, an alternative preventive use of enhancement genetic engineering can be imagined, such as altering the concentration of a protein that leads to heart disease. If the goal in this instance is the alleviation of disease, it may be ethically justified, representing a form of preventive medicine; the scientific situation would have to be clarified before this approach could be seriously contemplated.

Index

175